A DEN

Every year, 8500 people in the UK will have a subarachnoid haemorrhage, of whom about 50 per cent will survive this traumatic brain injury which often occurs without warning. Survivors can make a 'good' neurological recovery but the psychosocial impact can be longer lasting. Drawing from her own experience of surviving a subarachnoid haemorrhage, together with other people's journeys of recovery and recent research findings, Alison Wertheimer covers:

- themes of recovery
- leaving neurocare and early days of recovery
- looking for help
- physical, sensory and cognitive effects
- the emotional impact of subarachnoid haemorrhage
- the survivor's relationship with family and friends
- returning to work
- what helped the survivors with their recovery
- subarachnoid haemorrhage as a life-changing event.

A Dented Image will be of interest to a wide-ranging audience: survivors and their families and friends; health professionals working with people recovering from acute brain injury in hospital and community-based services including doctors, nurses, psychologists, physiotherapists, occupational therapists and other members of rehabilitation teams. It may also be of interest to people recovering from other traumatic illnesses or injuries.

Alison Wertheimer is a writer, researcher and counsellor. She is the author of *A Special Scar: The Experiences of People Bereaved by Suicide* (2001).

A DENTED IMAGE

Journeys of Recovery from Subarachnoid Haemorrhage

Alison Wertheimer

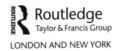

Routledge
Taylor & Francis Group

LONDON AND NEW YORK

First published 2008
by Routledge
27 Church Road, Hove, East Sussex, BN3 2FA

Simultaneously published in the USA and Canada
by Routledge

270 Madison Avenue, New York, NY 10016

Routledge is an imprint of the Taylor & Francis Group, an Informa business

Copyright © 2008 Alison Wertheimer

Typeset in Times by Garfield Morgan, Swansea, West Glamorgan
Printed and bound in Great Britain by TJ International Ltd, Padstow, Cornwall
Paperback cover design by Andy Ward

British Library Cataloguing in Publication Data
A catalogue record for this book is available from the British Library

Library of Congress Cataloging-in-Publication Data
Wertheimer, Alison.
A dented image : journeys of recovery from subarachnoid
haemorrhage / Alison Wertheimer.
p. ; cm.
Includes bibliographical references and index.
ISBN 978-0-415-38671-5 (hbk) – ISBN 978-0-415-38672-2 (pbk)
1. Subarachnoid haemorrhage–Patients–Interviews. 2. Subarachnoid
haemorrhage–Patients–Rehabilitation. 3. Subarachnoid
haemorrhage–Psychological aspects. I. Title.
[DNLM: 1. Subarachnoid Haemorrhage–psychology.
2. Subarachnoid Haemorrhage–rehabilitation. 3. Survivors–psychology.
WL 200 W499d 2008]
RC394.H37W48 2008
616.8'103–dc22
2008002881

ISBN: 978-0-415-38671-5 (hbk)
ISBN: 978-0-415-38672-2 (pbk)

I had underestimated how tightly the brain's functions are bound to the rest of the body, and, at the same time, how deeply they are embedded in the wider physical and social landscape. No brain is an island.

Broks, *Into the Silent Land*, 2003

I came to explore the wreck.
The words are purposes.
The words are maps.
I came to see the damage that was done
And the treasures that prevail.

Adrienne Rich, 'Diving into the Wreck'

CONTENTS

CONTENTS

PREFACE

This book had its genesis in May 2001 when I had a subarachnoid haemorrhage. After nearly a week of bad headaches, I was admitted to the National Hospital for Neurology and Neurosurgery via my local general hospital. About five weeks later, after two operations, and a second haemorrhage in between, I left hospital to begin the journey of recovery, unaware, at that time, what this might involve, or, indeed, how long the journey would last.

A few days after the first operation, I asked a friend to bring me in a notebook. At that stage my notes were fragmentary, but they acted as an aide memoire as well as an opportunity to record some initial reflections about what was happening. (Perhaps that's why I heard myself described by one of the nursing staff as 'the lady with the green notebook'.)

While spending a few days back at my local hospital before going home, another friend turned up with a large blue notebook, and suggested I wrote about my experiences. When that notebook was full, I graduated to my computer. I wrote a journal for the next two and a half years, after which the urge to write about all this seemed to be fading.

Towards the end of 2004 I showed my publisher some of the journals, though uncertain whether I wanted that degree of self-exposure or whether they would even be interested. Their suggestion that I interviewed fellow survivors, while including excerpts from my journals, sounded daunting, given my continuing mental fatigue and mild cognitive difficulties, but it would overcome my concerns about offering a single and purely personal perspective on recovery from subarachnoid haemorrhage.

So although the idea for writing a book about subarachnoid haemorrhage and recovery stemmed from personal experience, this final product is somewhat different, and, I hope, by shifting the focus to other survivors, this broader canvas will prove to be more useful. I have included extracts from my journals, and these appear as the Prologue.

Alison Wertheimer
February 2008

ACKNOWLEDGEMENTS

I would like to thank the following:

Mr Lawrence Watkins, consultant neurosurgeon, and staff at the National Hospital for Neurology and Neurosurgery whose skills and care made it possible for me to write this book.

Angela Collett, Carleen Scott and Sharon Swain of the Brain and Spine Foundation for their help and encouragement in the early stages of researching this book; and particular thanks to Angela Collett for reading the manuscript for medical accuracy and for offering general feedback.

Dr Issam Awad for permission to use the HSQuale Instrument on which I based the topic guide for the interviews; and Linda Jenkins for helpful comments on the guide.

Lesley Foulkes and Sarah Halcrow of the Wessex Neurological Centre, Southampton General Hospital, for putting me in touch with people willing to be interviewed and also to Lesley Foulkes for talking to me about the centre's Subarachnoid Haemorrhage and Cerebral Aneurysm Support Group.

Gerard Millsopp of the Val Hennessey Trust for putting me in touch with people willing to be interviewed.

Anne Rouse, who not only did a great job of transcribing the interviews, but also offered thoughtful comments and continuing support.

Eileen Campbell and Grace Kobbe for reading and commenting on some of the chapters.

Trevor Powell and David Jones who read the final manuscript.

My editor, Joanne Foreshaw, at Brunner-Routledge, for continuing support and encouragement.

Geshe Tashi Tsering and Jamyang Buddhist Centre, for offering refuge in recovery.

My very special thanks to the survivors who welcomed me into their homes and shared their experiences of recovery with me and with the readers of this book.

Above all, I want to express my very deep gratitude to friends and family who supported me through my long journey of recovery, particularly those whose steadfast presence helped me through the dark days. I am not naming them individually but I hope they know who they are.

Permissions

The lines from 'Diving into the Wreck'. Copyright © 2002 by Adrienne Rich. Copyright © 1973 by W.W. Norton & Company, Inc. from THE FACT OF A DOORFRAME: SELECTED POEMS 1950–2001 by Adrienne Rich. Used by permission of the author and W.W. Norton & Company Inc.

The lines from 'Jigsaw' on pp. 238–9, by Mark Ward, published in *The Friend*, 24 August 2001, p. 12.

The Brain and Spine Foundation and Wessex Neurocare for the Glossary of Terms in Appendix D.

The lines from *Into the Silent Land*. Copyright © Paul Broks 2003. Used by permission of the author and Atlantic Books.

Dr Jan Wallcraft for permission to quote from 'Turning towards recovery: a study of personal narratives of mental health crisis and breakdown'. PhD dissertation, South Bank University, London.

PROLOGUE

A brief word of explanation here about the 'dented image'. During the second operation, a bone flap (a part of my skull) was removed and replaced in a third operation four months later. During this time, my head had a rather large dent. As I also soon realised, my self-image and self-confidence were also dented. Now there is only a minimal physical indentation but it took somewhat longer to repair that psychological dent.

Having decided to include a brief account of my experiences of recovery, using extracts from my journals, when it came to it, deciding what to include was much more difficult than I'd anticipated. Personal accounts of coping with illness are appearing in bookshops more and more frequently with their readership apparently extending beyond those directly affected. However, it seemed easier to write here about other people's experiences than to share my own. Why was this so?

Looking back at what I had written, I find it hard to discern my reasons for doing so. There are certainly many pages which form a litany of woe – the germs of a misery memoir? On other days I was listing my most recent achievements, presumably to encourage myself – a 'you *can* recover from a brain haemorrhage' approach but perhaps subsequently *pour encourager les autres*?

As I struggled with whether or not to include 'my story', I came across an article on medical narratives which seemed to address my dilemma:

> Michael Blastland: Talking about illness isn't only a selfish fascination . . . but it's also a way of turning something that could take you down a sink of introspection into something more open and engaged and curious.

1

> Francesca Happé: It's so personal that it seems wrong to share it, yet at the same time you have this enormous connection with other people in the same situation
>
> (Blastland *et al.* 2007: 48)

I didn't want to end up producing what have sometimes been dubbed 'misery memoirs' or 'sick lit'. On the other hand, I didn't want to gloss over the difficult times and produce a work of 'how I triumphed over adversity'. I hope that what appears here (and in the rest of the book) transmits a more mixed and hopefully realistic message: subarachnoid haemorrhage is a shocking and traumatic event and recovery can be difficult and, at times, very hard work, but if life changes as a result, then those changes can also be positive. There are losses to be mourned and gains to be celebrated. I have tried to strike a balance.

The interviews with survivors in this book were conversations, allowing time and space for reflection and hindsight, but journal writing is something quite other. At the time, I wrote with no audience in mind – except myself. Now, I've toyed with the idea of adding, or updating what I wrote, but have decided to leave what I wrote without embellishment or further explanation.

I have taken the liberty of altering my journals in one respect. After the first six months, I started writing in the third person ['She . . . she . . .] but now I've changed this to the first person. Why? Perhaps because at that stage of recovery, I was trying to distance myself from what was actually happening, because life was often so difficult. Now it's time to reclaim those 'stories' as 'my stories'.

I wrote the journals while recovering from an acute brain injury, despite hearing the doctors' opining that I was 'neurologically intact'. Now I'm able to spot 'errors', missing words, occasional inconsistencies. If they are evident, both here and elsewhere in this book, please attribute them to my largely healed but still recovering brain.

MAY 2000? (UNDATED)

Vivid memories – dreams? – in the early days: taking part in a bank robbery at Elephant and Castle – being attacked by strangers – walls in the sitting room and kitchen in my flat all unsafe and bulging.

Some strong visual memories around first and second operations. G at bottom left [of my bed] looking very worried and another time A at bottom right looking rather shocked by my black eye.

Nearly everyone wants you to have a 'speedy' recovery – how can I explain that this *won't* be very speedy?

16 JUNE 2001

D [a friend] explained: first operation was fine and they did a bone resection but then I was bleeding, so they had to do further surgery late pm; bleeding inside the skull and pressure built up inside and had to open skull to relieve the pressure – 'subdural haematoma'.

Bad evening – nausea and some headache . . . the impact of my 'near miss' after the first operation beginning to hit home? Eventually slept from about 11 pm to 5.30 am – an unbroken sleep as though I needed to shut down for a few hours.

20 JUNE 2001

Nearer to getting home – nervous . . . S [a nurse] washed my hair in the shower – great! . . . replaces my bandage . . . this time tomorrow I'll be home – feels *very* strange but getting home is an important transition.

21 JUNE 2001

[Early morning] Lie and think about the flat and wonder if it'll be okay. I know it's about confidence in myself. [Later] Stepped into the flat about 5 pm – overwhelmed by sense of peace. G arrived about 7 pm and we had quiet time – talk, delicious supper – *bliss*.

29 JUNE 2001

C [friend and neighbour] has really come up trumps – washed my hair and let me touch 'it' [the dent] when I felt I could – and left me when I didn't look and couldn't. She drew [a picture] and explained 'it' – which must have a name soon. . . . found two possible sources of hats on mail order. . . phone call from the hospital – [bicycle] helmet to be worn (except in bed) all the time until doctors' review on 30 July. It's uncomfortable and unsightly but it seems orders are orders.

30 JUNE 2001

Had to will myself to get out of bed and put [the helmet] on – lots of thoughts in the night about disfigurement and the 'dented image' . . . I'm crying and mourning the 'undented' me . . . I can't always be a good/perfect patient and I can't always cope – superwoman has taken a knock.

1 JULY 2001

Talking to J, I've realised how squeamish and afraid some people have been about hospital visits . . . I wonder what they thought they'd see – ET in bed? A vegetable? Someone who would no longer be me? How powerful our fantasies are around the brain and its 'insults'!

5 JULY 2001

Probably the most difficult day so far . . . Feeling 'why me?' and 'it's not fair – hard to accept what has happened as just life. But positively – two weeks at home and I'm okay. Started having baths this week and hospital today says I'm not having to wear a helmet.

10 JULY 2001

This is a tale of woe – I feel I'm being very self-pitying . . . everyone else seems to be getting on with their lives and I can feel quite angry and envious of them. It's not just 'depression', inertia, heaviness – it's often real crying, tears, misery.

12 JULY 2001

Be patient! It's less than two months since the aneurysm started [to bleed].

13 JULY 2001

What kind of lady of leisure am I at the moment? . . . Start of the weekend for some people, the reward of 'free time' for a week's work – time (and money) earned but what have I earned? A year off work – a gift? Can it ever get to feel like a gift? It feels more of a punishment at the moment.

15 JULY 2001

Remind myself that I *have* coped with very little medical/ nursing support from anyone. It was *me* who wrote to [my GP] and got nurses to prescribe dressings, *me* who tried to get advice from the hospital; *no* GP contact for two months.

19 JULY 2001

I *hate* having to be so dependent.

20 JULY 2001

This is so like bereavement – the ebb and flow, the back and forth from coping to non-coping, and the tears.

25 JULY 2001

Remember! It's only just over one month since I left hospital and if it's a year's recovery [since the haemorrhage], I've (only) done two and a half months.

1 AUGUST 2001

Two more emails – 'Don't know how serious this is' . . . 'hope you're enjoying life at home' – leave me feeling angry and sending rather sharp rejoinders. How can people think it's minor or enjoyable when I've lost so much and life often feels like an unending series of losses and struggles just to manage day-to-day life. Maybe I should just stay shtum and not comment at all? But I feel a bit better and maybe people should be educated more about this whole business? I certainly wasn't.

4 AUGUST 2001

Some of this really mirrors a bereavement – most mornings when I wake up I've forgotten where I'm at now – with my dented head – after a few seconds a cloud of (faint) depression descends and I'm so full of, overwhelmed by, my situation – the pain, the loss, the struggles, but then I get up and potter around and enjoy the first cup of real coffee. Enjoy the smaller pleasures – look at small things which can delight.

6 AUGUST 2001

Tired and weepy (especially the latter) today – but lovely woman at the [Brain and Spine Foundation] helpline who I rang to ask about yoga, was so nice and understanding when I burst into tears and said this was a bad day – as though the tears are dammed up in between when I feel I'm doing okay; but I don't want pills – it's got to be 'wept through'; but she said you'll be tired for up to (at least) six months and people have good and bad days – also said to me what a difference the next operation [my bone flap replacement] will make – restoring my image to some extent?

12 AUGUST 2001

Shaky time – headache started early yesterday evening – got very panicky but eventually slept . . . fantasies of everything repeating . . . trying to calm down and not spin off into future possible scenarios [of readmission returning to hospital, etc.].

20 AUGUST 2001

In my ninth week at home and the main theme is 'waiting' for the operation date for the National [hospital]. Trying not to idealise it as the answer to everything – my head may not be quite the shape I want it to be *but* I'll have to learn to live with that? – and be a hat wearer.

24 AUGUST 2001

A first! Washed my own hair, watched and supervised by C. I *can* achieve.

26 AUGUST 2001

Snakes and ladders? I've just hit the snake on the board?

28 AUGUST 2001

Awful night. . . . I think all the impact of trauma in late May is now surging . . . I think I've coped until now but the coping resources aren't infinite. What must I hear, accept and live with: Death is part of life and inevitable; things like my SAH can happen very suddenly and totally unexpectedly – out of the blue; I can't control everything that happens to me – all this wasn't on my agenda. Am I too easily hooked into being a 'good patient' and a 'coper'? Don't other people need to know – be told by me – that I'm *not* coping at times? Is this delayed shock? Don't talk airily to people about my 'brain haemorrhage' etc. and the fact that I nearly died.

4 SEPTEMBER 2001

What's difficult? No operation date. Post-traumatic stress? Feeling I'm struggling on my own. Coping strategies depleted after 11 weeks from leaving Queen Square [hospital]. No [incapacity] benefit.

What's on my side? A lot of good and constant friends; some friends who *do* understand; family who care – in their own way; I've *survived* all this trauma. My brain is still working.

13 SEPTEMBER 2001

A roller-coaster day – a haircut at last and G [an elderly friend] died early this morning. Feel glad I had a haircut; sensible thing to do though felt quite anxious in the salon but it feels so much better and J [my hairdresser] was *so* nice.

18 SEPTEMBER 2001

Still feeling very anxious and panicky . . . general sense of being very vulnerable – the world being unsafe and unpredictable. Anxiety about going back to hospital? After a difficult, anxiety-filled day indoors, here are some positives: I'm 'neurologically intact'; I'm alive; I've got good and caring friends; I've coped on my own; I'm financially okay.

Why might I be weary/exhausted? Since coming home 13 weeks ago, I've had 81 visits from people, including giving a meal to 23 people, been out for a meal with 12 people; washing, ironing, shopping, paperwork, nominal housework.

7 OCTOBER 2001

Talking with D and other friends is an opportunity to 'talk out' some of the huge amount of reflecting and thinking through which this has thrown at me.

9 OCTOBER 2001

Stitches out! Yes, my head is 'scarred' but it's mine. Feel rather relieved that [my GP] wants me to use a dressing for another two weeks to flatten the scar. . . . Washed and dried my hair which felt a lot better and I felt I'd reclaimed something of myself. Wept.

8

PROLOGUE

15 OCTOBER 2001

What a bummer. Walking along, suddenly developed tinnitus in my right ear which is *very* hard to tolerate. Contacted Tinnitus Action who have a very reassuring phone message – asked them to send info.

16 OCTOBER 2001

You and Yours [radio programme] is debating euthanasia but I realise how much potential/actual life I have – I can eat, walk, go out, talk, control my bodily functions; that's not a bad list.

17 OCTOBER 2001

The days seem to lack a structure – am I now a 'lady who lunches' on some days; too much focus on being a conva- lescent but no operations to face, just outpatient appointments and neuropathic pain, tinnitus and sometimes a lack of energy and creativity. What to do to give my life more focus? Shape? Meaning? Hard to fix goals when the future – even 2002 – seems so nebulous.

20 NOVEMBER 2001

I'm *bored* with too much leisure – this doesn't mean that I don't like any leisure – socialising, reading, etc. but there's too much of it at the moment . . . Too much of a sameness and this isn't a normal lifestyle – even if I had retired – not that that is on my agenda at the moment!

5 JANUARY 2002

Maybe by committing myself to writing every day . . . is the only thing at present where I feel I 'can do'. Standing in the kitchen earlier this morning – . . . I thought to call this a diary *of* despair but then I found myself thinking – call this a diary *through* despair.

9

I start each day with a faint tinge of optimism ' the 'all will be well'-ness of Eliot and Julian of Norwich, but that dissipates as though there is a dragon which creeps out of its lair and opens its mouth to belch what(?) over me. Where does that image come from? Is it part of the huge anger . . . that makes me go round the flat or lie in bed muttering . . . sh*t, sh*t, sh*t, or even f**ck, f**k, f**k. . . . feeling that life will never be better, no one will ever want or need me to do anything for them?

What am I committed to doing to try and make things different for myself? Writing a page of this journal every day. Having the courage to hold a belief in the future? Write about other than despair. (NOW: I can hear birds singing; the house feels peaceful and quiet; I have almost got through sorting out the filing cabinet though it can't be in nice neat colour-coded categories because life isn't that neat or clear at the moment.)

6 JANUARY 2002

I can't wait to get my car back at the end of March [or early April] − [it] seems to have become a symbol of independence, of steering my own course, being in control of something again; at least I hope I will feel in control.

The flat [has] come to embody much of what I feel about myself − run down, needing renewal and more TLC [tender loving care].

7 JANUARY 2002

This really is the deadest time of the year. What to write about today? I have no desire, no energy, no sense of movement as though there is nothing worth doing which gives me pleasure . . . Operation sites have been intermittently tight or a bit painful.

Today is the major return to work and I sit here so aware that I have no 'work' to return to. I hated P's Christmas card enjoining me to take a holiday, to rest, to take things very easy or carefully. I could scream at people: let me have my life back pleeeeeeeeease. However tiring it was − or will be − I want to be productive.

What have I done here on this page today, except express my general boredom, hatred of others for having a life. Rebuilding a post-SAH life is turning out to be *so* much harder than I anticipated. My fine – deluded? – ideas in the hospital were so far from the hard reality of trying to shape something new. An image has finally appeared: the potter's clay which waits to be shaped into 'something new' but I just want to punch the clay.

11 JANUARY 2002

I wonder what happened to the time when I nearly died but of which I have so few memories: G at the end of the bed – a distant voice talking about a 'second operation'; A looking appalled with her hand over her mouth; an Irish nurse must have been trying to rouse me and I said, rather irritably. 'Leave me alone.' . . . Where did those memories go? Where and how can they resurface? Will they resurface? Will it be like the sheer fear, panic and 'nameless dread' of Bion? What a wonderful term . . . but so very unpleasant.

13 JANUARY 2002

! was standing at the bus stop in Moorgate when the driver pulled up at the traffic lights opposite. I'd been to M&S which, rather disconcertingly, had mirrors everywhere and the sight (site?) of my still rather cropped head didn't do much for my self-esteem. I didn't feel great about my image, but didn't have a good 'feeling' about this man in an oldish red saloon with his mates.

'Oi,' he called out. I wondered what he would say next. Swiftly I realised he wasn't going to ask directions to some-where. I had a bad feel about this. 'You're the ugliest person I've ever seen,' he called – presumably for his mates' benefit? Were they all laughing. A kind of 'verbal vandalism' perhaps? A sort of unprovoked 'road rage' since I wasn't even behind the wheel of my car.

I stood silently; ashamed, feeling myself to be ugly, won-dering whether to walk across and tell him about the brain haemorrhage. I wanted to stun him into silence; I didn't want to shame him; I wanted him to be understanding, nice, apologetic. The traffic lights changed to green and the car moved away . . . I felt tears welling up.

16 JANUARY 2002

Borderland. I have felt myself to be 'at the border'. After all, a person who is at the border belongs neither to one country nor the other. Perhaps I am a citizen of nowhere? . . . Now I feel I'm in neither one place nor the other although I remember in past times I'd been one of those worker-ants, worker-bees. . . . let me join you, let me come and take part in that life you have. I want to be one of the normals, though if a year ago someone had told me I'd be in another country for many months, I would have said great, wonderful, just what I always wanted to do.

At first, in the hospital, I had been content to remain in Sick-Land. . . . But then I moved to Sick-Land-At-Home and the flat which had always felt a place I dashed into and out of in my busy life became a prison. It was for many weeks the place where visitors from Well-Land came freely across the border to see me but they could always leave Sick-Land behind.

I need others to tell me that 'acute brain injury' doesn't mean my brain is permanently damaged. Earlier today when I made the calculation error about the chocolate, I felt yet again that tightness, that fear that when I did go back to work I would make awful mistakes.

18 JANUARY 2002

Until I actually have a piece of work in my hands, it's difficult to predict how things will go. I'm worried that there will be some cognitive problems. Getting muddled with recipes, getting on to the wrong branch of the Northern Line − these and other little mistakes prey on my mind . . . mistakes will occur and when they do, as they surely will, it's important not to see them as a total disaster or decide that they're conclusive proof that I'm permanently brain damaged.

PROLOGUE

29 JANUARY 2002

I can hear myself becoming easily bored and frustrated as I recount the 'story of my illness' over and over again. This happens quite often at the moment when I'm networking with people who I haven't seen or talked with since last May. It's become a story – as though I'm talking about a stranger.

5 FEBRUARY 2002

Is Judith Herman right when she writes in *Trauma and Recovery* about the need to reconnect with the world as being one of the tasks or stages in recovery?

My head has also been quite 'tight' and a constant remember of what happened with all those operations last year. My body is not in a very healing or healed state at the moment and that builds on my anxiety about recovery and fears about whether I will ever recover.

I liked the descriptive information about the [Buddhist] Peace Garden and the six 'perfections' – of generosity, diligence, patience, discipline, concentration and wisdom.

6 FEBRUARY 2002

You can't go back to being exactly the same person as you were before the trauma happened; neither can you carry on with the same assumptions. I have to learn to accept that I'm not invincible; that my body – my healthy functioning – can let me down.

How do you find out if you're brain damaged? I don't know anything about brains! But I CAN accept that things like the nerve twinges and pains in my right arm after the third operation have healed now. Only now very occasionally does my thumb of my right hand tingle or go numb.

How strange . . . I'd completely forgotten that [after leaving school] I'd worked in Germany in a neurosurgical clinic. But I know that whenever I walked through Queen Square and read that notice – The National Hospital for Neurosurgery and Neurology – I would shudder and avert my eyes. And yet now it was my 'home' for over five weeks and the place where I now walk in, know my way around and feel I belong.

I know and can really appreciate [or sort of] that everyone wants things to be better for me. How can I pretend when inside things are so bleak.

7 FEBRUARY 2002

A bad night last night – boiling hot and neuropathically painful legs and feet.

I'm aware when I go out these days how so little pleases my senses. I remember when I first came out of hospital how I felt my face was frozen in a rather rigid way of no smiles and little laughter. I wonder now if it was about the muscle on that side of my face having been cut during surgery?

But is that lack of oomph in my senses also related in some way to the numbness in my head – though I can now touch those bits of my skull which are not where the bone flap is sited. Am I sure that I can now feel a bit more of a normal sense on my head – towards the back – where there has been numbness until recently. The hospital's handout says your skull can be numb for up to a year or so, so maybe they are right.

9 FEBRUARY 2002

Clothes are a problem at the moment . . . I'm wearing far too much black at the moment . . . I've thrown out loads of clothes since last May but now I can't engage with what I *do* want to wear. It's as though I don't know what I want to present to the world?

Be kind to yourself about things like weight and clothes – all part and parcel of the same thing. Be generous about how you are. Don't slap on more critical thoughts about being fat and sloppy. Allow yourself time to get better from a virus and a bad back – oh, and three neurosurgical procedures in the last nine months.

Go out into the sunshine. Breathe some good fresh air . . . Go and sit and drink a latte somewhere too!

14

17 FEBRUARY 2002

A friend mailed me a story yesterday about how Itzhak Perlman's violin string broke but rather than going offstage to get a new string with all the palaver of his [physical] disability, he managed to play and perform brilliantly with the remaining three strings. The first time I read this through I felt (a) resentful that someone was trying to cheer me up and (b) didn't want to 'play on three strings'. I thought I wanted four strings or nothing. BUT is this part of what I'm struggling with now. Do I feel that it has to be all or nothing? Or is there a message for me in that story that actually I am playing pretty well on three strings at the moment – at least that is what most people see.

What helps and what hurts?

It hurts: when I'm awake in the middle of the night and can't get back to sleep; when I 'make a mistake' – like forgetting my specs when going to the theatre last Monday – and then feeling very stupid and, worse, worrying that I'm seriously cognitively impaired; when I lose sight of all the progress and hard work I have put into recovering over the last nine months.

It helps: when I'm in the company of other people that I enjoy; when I can recognise and really know that it will take time and patience to recover; when I'm in contact with people who knew/ know me as Alison – a successful self-employed person; when I keep going rather than turn to magic pills to cure the depression . . . Remember the people in my life who *are* there for me so much of the time and who are willing me to recover.

AUGUST 2002

Some of the losses I've experienced have included:

- an illusion that I was immortal
- an illusion that I could work 24/7 without looking after myself and without any ill-effects
- not being able to drive for nearly a year and not being able to be 'at the steering wheel'
- huge loss of self-confidence and self-esteem
- finding it difficult or impossible to make large or small decisions

- not being able to work so not having a lot of positive feedback
- not having the security of earning money
- loss of my identity and role as a counsellor
- loss of my work with and links with King's.

Some of these were temporary losses (e.g. I'm driving again and working) and some are maybe permanent – a part of me?

Some of the gains or learning (though not all consolidated!) include:

- working towards a better work–life balance
- seeing more movies, going to more exhibitions, etc.
- learning some meditation/relaxation practices
- reading much more than I used to
- thinking more, thinking things through, not just shooting from the hip
- thinking things through so that sometimes even with basic 'living' (e.g. programming my new radio) I feel a sense of mastery/achievement
- having made some new friends or some acquaintances have become friends
- making more time to see friends (rather than saying I was too busy-busy)
- generally slowing down (a bit) and not doing everything at 100 mph
- thinking more – when feeling was always my superior function . . . so not rushing around or into things but being more thoughtful.

23 AUGUST 2002

It's 11 months since my last operation and I can see that I've come a long way since then.

18 SEPTEMBER 2002

Last appointment with Mr Watkins ['my' consultant neuro-surgeon]. Need to remind myself how far I've come in the six months since I last saw Mr Watkins. The pain/hotness in my feet is much better; I haven't had pins and needles that much recently; my head is a lot less tight and sore and I can go for periods of time without really being too aware of the bone flap area. AND the depression is a lot better than it was even when I went to the pain clinic just over two months ago, I recently threw away the hospital phone number and address which I carried round with me in my purse so I'm able to let go of that now. Shook hands and left with smiles on both sides. Went to the West End; had a celebratory coffee and an almond and cherry croissant and saw a good film.

A friend says, 'You're now back to your old self.' But I'm not my old self as I slightly crossly pointed out. I'm a different self – a re-covered self even . . . there are people who want me to be back to the old Alison . . . How can they want the old me back? I like this new/changed me much better! Why do people want to get you back to where you were?

For more or less the first time I find myself writing 'I think' rather than always writing 'I feel . . .'. Strange that it took me to have a brain haemorrhage for my brain to work better!

4 OCTOBER 2002

I have been interviewed by [an employee assistance provider] about counselling work and they'd like me to do the sessions! I started my French class last night and although I was very nervous and didn't perform brilliantly I was probably average in a very mixed ability group of about 12 people. I had a really enjoyable lunch with [a colleague] . . . and she asked whether I'd be intererested in any future work. I've lost 2 lb weight.

7 OCTOBER 2002

I still have difficulties with that period after the first operation and until just after the second operation. I have no conscious-ness of that time that can be rediscovered and thought about. I'm left with a gap. The visits in hospital from a senior psy-chologist and from Judy Watkin were really too soon. I was in a

17

very shocked and dissociated state and couldn't take in what they were saying but now I want to try and remember what I was told.

21 OCTOBER 2002

Decided to get out into the sunshine . . . to [Hampstead] Heath . . . absolutely glorious. Several months ago it might have felt less good . . . blue blue skies and autumn foliage.

1 NOVEMBER 2002

Relationships . . . continue to be a difficulty . . . there are maybe several strands to think about: I'm not the huge centre of attention and concern that I was last year when I was in hospital and in the first few weeks or even months; I'm a much more 'thinking' and 'analytical' person these days and so have a different 'take' on some relationships and these tend to be the ones I find difficult. I'm perhaps less 'generous' but more realistic about the give and take of many relationships.

Lots of negative thoughts and preoccupations around at the moment so I'm going to make myself *think* about some achievements in the last few days:

21 NOVEMBER 2002

This week my feet have started 'revving up' again at night (and a bit yesterday evening before bedtime) and the bone flap area has hurt a bit, particularly when I'm tired but also need to remember that cold weather affects old 'breaks' or fractures which was what happened to my skull.

25 NOVEMBER 2002

I'm so tired I really can't think straight, write anything that's very useful so be kind to yourself, cherish yourself and just leave this until there is a moment for writing more.

13 JANUARY 2003

Looking back over the time of recovery I think there's been a lot of travel down different roads and some of them could be seen as 'false starts' – but maybe there's more to some of those things than just 'negatives'? I may not have found I want to stay with some people/places/things but maybe they were stepping stones as I navigated a river – not quite the image I'm looking for but I know I am the kind of person who has 'enthusiasms' in terms of picking things up and running with them for a time and then turning to something else.

I think I'm maybe caught up in trying to build a perfect path to recovery with some very clear, definite and even quite large building bricks. It may be more useful to see them as smaller stones . . . all different shapes and sizes and maybe sometimes they need to be regrouped or have things added?

18 JANUARY 2003

Heard myself saying to several people recently that if I thought I was working hard before the SAH then this is at times even more hard work but it's a different kind of work. I feel as though I have to construct and shape my life in a much more proactive way.

Offers of work started hotting up this week . . . Of course I'm relieved that I can feel a bit more financially secure but I think there's more to it than just, wow, I can occupy myself.

Didn't know what I wanted to do when I woke up this morning; there's a new proof-read which in the 'old days' I would have leapt up and started to work on but now I don't feel the same way. I'm sitting here writing this instead and I walked down to the market, wishing that I could have walked more and further. . . .

Concentration is quite a problem at the moment . . . What ideas do I have? Avoid multitasking (what is seen in our day and age as a virtue seems to run counter to mindfulness). Do I need to have the radio playing all the time? At least go for music rather than voices? When I'm engaged in something, then my mind says, why don't you do something else, make a note if necessary but don't leap up and make a phone call, for example. Stay focused.

What are now the things that seem to really help me?

- walking – definitely gets a lot of votes
- journalling – I mostly enjoy doing this and even if I never go back and read all this then I have a way of reviewing things (literally sometimes) and the jottings between writing on the computer can be useful
- spending more time with friends, even though this fluctuates as their lives fluctuate in busyness (and mine when work is coming in)
- getting out of bed at a more or less fixed time – not enjoyable, but helpful
- meditation (sort of and some days) and mindfulness of breathing
- monthly massage or reflexology sessions
- exploring a Buddhist approach to living: trying to be more mindful and remembering the six perfections.

15 FEBRUARY 2003

The sun is shining brightly at 9 o'clock after a week of grey skies . . . One way and another it's been a full week, with some occasionally difficult moments but I feel right now a sense of achievement – of achievements?

Reclaiming weekends: I could do a couple of hours work before going to meet [friends] but I'm really beginning to get a sense of weekends these days – a feeling that the week has a different shape – a 5 + 2 rather than a 7 (or 24/7). I'm starting to look forward to weekends with a sense of anticipation. Perhaps because there's plenty of work to do Monday–Fridays but it's about the *use of time* and wanting to do different and enjoyable/pleasurable things on Saturdays and Sundays.

Spent most of this week editing the working document [on children with disabilities, for the Department of Health] which has turned out to be rather more awful and complex than I envisaged. Some moments of panic, depression, feeling useless but I ploughed on and did four days . . . I think my speed of work is improving a bit and with this I was able to stand back and really evaluate what was me (finding the task pretty difficult) and what was them (a pig's eye of a document – sorry pigs).

4 MARCH 2003

Journalling seems to go in fits and starts. Some bursts of energetic writing last month and then a bit of a gap.

Things aren't the same now as two years ago. I'm trying to live my life differently. To be slower, not to multitask and rush around like a blue-arsed fly doing far too many jobs and trying to hold it all together.

12 MAY 2003

I sat down to start writing this three days before coming here [for final session of CBT and final visit to the hospital].

Many years ago, I used to drink at the Queen's Larder pub (and on one memorable occasion managed to lock myself in the ladies' loo). I always noticed the hospital and hoped I'd never need to go through its doors. Now when I walk through the square, I have very mixed feelings and I know that this hospital will always have some importance for me, even though the feelings will fade over time. I think I'll always retain an affection for the National.

When I typed NHNN on the computer just now my spell-check came up with several alternatives including 'nanny' which seemed quite appropriate. The hospital has felt like a nanny at times – mostly a rather kind, caring and benign one – but when you grow up you leave your nanny behind (or most people do).

I will always be grateful to the people here who saved my life when I re-bled after the first operation. Coming to terms with what happened that week has been very hard and I still find it odd that I remember so little of that time but I'm so glad that I did survive.

So I leave here knowing that my life has changed – probably more and in more different ways than anything else that has happened to me before. I think in the last two years I've had some of the worst times in my whole life, but I know that I've also gained more than ever before.

Part I

SETTING THE SCENE

1

BACKGROUND

Every year, 8500 people in the UK will have a subarachnoid haemorrhage (a leakage of blood over the surface of the brain) – that's about one person every hour. Of those 8500 people about half will survive. This book is about some of their experiences and their journeys of recovery. Subarachnoid haemorrhage is an acute brain injury, so we start by looking at what our brains may mean to us.

What do our brains mean to us?

Despite the comparatively recent upsurge of interest in the workings of the brain by neuroscientists, neuropsychologists and other researchers (and a Google search of 'brain' currently produces over 153 million entries), unless we have a professional interest in matters of the brain, most of us don't spend a great deal of time wondering what's going on beneath our skull, and what our brain is getting up to.

The people whose experiences are recounted here hadn't usually spent much time dwelling on what their brain was doing; they generally took it for granted. Seven months after his brain haemorrhage, David said: 'You know you've got an aching knee – oh dear! – But you forget about your brain.' Like David, Pam also hadn't particularly focused on her brain:

I'm not sure it meant anything to me. I mean, people used to say 'Oh, you've got a good brain', and I think I took pride in my ability to use my brain to think creatively, to be articulate; I say, I took pride in it, but it wasn't something I felt incredibly aware of . . . it was just part of who I am.

And Kaz echoed this:

> I suppose it wasn't until after [the haemorrhage] happened,
> then you think, oh my God! . . . I mean your brain is a really
> important part of you . . . after what happened to me you think
> what could have happened so, yeah, you do take it for granted.
> You don't realise it's one of your major organs, really.

So we may take our brains for granted, but trying to understand
what the brain actually means and how it operates isn't easy either.
Perhaps we're more likely to be aware of our 'head' rather than our
'brain'. Even though she's a trained nurse, after her brain haemorrhage Wendy found that: 'When you used to get a headache, you
don't think "my brain is hurting"; it's just your head. . . . there's
something in there but it's almost like it's not really there . . . it's
still not very tangible.'

As the neuropsychologist Paul Broks writes: 'To look at any
brain is to confront a deep mystery' (2003: 117). Asked what their
brain meant to them after their haemorrhage, survivors described it
variously as 'the most powerful part of us', 'the control panel of the
whole body', or 'the most delicate part of your body'. So perhaps
our brains can seem very strong but at the same time potentially
very vulnerable.

For others, their brain defined who they were. In one person's
words, it is 'who you are', and for another, 'from the neck up, is
me'; a repository for 'memory', 'taste', and 'thoughts'. Lesley
Foulkes, specialist nurse at the Wessex Neurological Centre, would
agree: 'Your brain is what makes you who you are.'

After his haemorrhagic stroke, Robert McCrum wrote: '[The
brain] weighs only 1.4 kilograms and yet it defines our whole
personality and our interaction with the world' (1998: 42–3). And
for Claudia Osborn, who sustained a major head injury, the brain
is 'the very engine, guidance system and repository of a person's
mind, experiences and personality' (1998: ix).

So these are some of the manifold meanings of the brain for
people who have sustained an acute brain injury, but what does it
mean to neurosurgeons – the 'brain surgeons' – who get to see and
touch people's brains? The stereotype of a brain surgeon is usually
of someone who is clever – even rather brainy. (Question: What do
you want to be when you grow up? Answer: A brain surgeon.) The
neurosurgeon's skills and knowledge are critical when someone is

operated on for a brain haemorrhage, but do they see beyond the 'grey matter'? For neurosurgeon Henry Marsh, it sometimes felt 'as though I was holding a human soul in my hands' (BBC 2004). And Neil Kitchen finds that when 'you just see the brain sitting there, that is that person, that human' (Guardian 2007). Whether or not we believe in the existence of the soul, it's an attractive idea:

> It feels natural to believe that something like a soul exists
> . . . We all feel that as well as a brain, something else
> occupies the interior of our head and the heads of other
> people – an irreducible mental core, the origin of thought
> and actions. It is a primitive belief, but it is compelling.
> (Broks 2003: 61)

So we ascribe many different meanings to the space beneath the skull, but when something totally unexpected and life threatening happens in that space, such as a subarachnoid haemorrhage, it's no wonder we find this deeply unsettling. If another part of our body is injured, 'we have this way of separating ideas of "the person" from what is happening to "the person's body"' (Broks 2003: 62–3). When our brain defines who we are, then separateness really isn't possible.

The following sections explain the reasons why this book was written, the sources which have been used to provide a range of perspectives on brain haemorrhage and the contents of the remaining chapters.

Why this book was written

The starting point for this book was my own experience of having a subarachnoid haemorrhage in 2001 and the journey of recovery which followed it, but aside from my personal narrative I have drawn on the experiences of fellow survivors (see Chapter 3), providing a much fuller and richer picture of the impact of having a brain haemorrhage and how they found their way through recovery. By describing their experiences here, perhaps this will lessen the isolation commonly experienced by other survivors.

No two people's recovery will be identical, but despite the differences similarities also emerge – not only in the ways in which the haemorrhage affected people's lives, but in the ways they coped with psychological and social recovery. The physical effects of subarachnoid haemorrhage are also described (see Chapter 7), but mainly because of their psychological and social impact.

A further aim of this book is to explore some of the currently unmet needs amongst survivors and their families. The very brief list of support groups (see Appendix C) and the under-provision of specialist nurses highlight the need to improve the support which survivors receive after leaving specialist hospital care. Although this book has not been written as a definitive manual for recovery, I have signposted sources of information, advice and support (see Appendix B).

A word about words

The language of subarachnoid haemorrhage

Writing this book has raised some interesting issues of language and at times I found it difficult to decide which terms to use. As Chapter 2 will discuss, it is not always clear whether subarachnoid haemorrhage is an 'illness', an 'injury', or an 'accident'. Chapter 4 considers whether 'recovery' or 'progress' best describes what happens after a haemorrhage. But how do we describe those directly affected? Are they 'patients', 'sufferers', or perhaps 'survivors'? The latter term is one I have discussed elsewhere in relation to a completely different group of people (Wertheimer 2001) but I am going to use the same term here. Half of those who have a subarachnoid haemorrhage will die, either immediately or shortly afterwards. The people whose experiences are described here are indeed survivors, so this is how I have chosen to refer to them. (Writing about women's experiences of haemorrhagic stroke, Sharon Dale Stone also explains why she made the same choice (Stone 2007: 21.)

A range of perspectives

I have drawn on a number of different sources which offer a variety of perspectives, but my starting point and the main focus of this book has been the interviews with 27 survivors. In addition, there are three written accounts and some of those who were interviewed also made available what they had written about their experiences. I have also included extracts from other individual narratives of recovery from brain haemorrhage, notably those by the actress Jane Lapotaire (2003) and the writer Robert McCrum (1998).

Jane Lapotaire describes her work *Time Out of Mind* (2003) as 'an attempt to explain to myself what happened in the days and months that followed [a ruptured aneurysm] . . . an attempt to describe the journey to recovery' and the challenge of getting to know a stranger, namely herself.

In *My Year Off: Rediscovering Life After a Stroke* (1998), Robert McCrum describes his recovery from a severe haemorrhagic stroke at the age of 42. Aimed partly at helping others who have suffered 'an insult to the brain' and their carers, he was also writing 'as a way to make sense of an extraordinary personal upheaval whose consequences will be with me until I die'.

More recently, Sharon Dale Stone has published a collection of women's stories of haemorrhagic stroke, *A Change of Plans*, focusing on gender perspectives, but also raising issues around recovery and rehabilitation, self-image, relationships with family, friends and work colleagues, and stroke as a life-changing experience (2007). Brief accounts of individual experiences of recovery can also be found in a paper about a study by Jarvis (2002) who interviewed eight people 14 to 18 months after their brain haemorrhage.

During my own recovery and while researching this book, I came across personal accounts by people recovering from other injuries or illnesses which, I felt, offered insights relevant to recovery from brain haemorrhage so they have been included. Two examples follow. The neurologist Oliver Sacks has written extensively about his patients, but in *A Leg To Stand On* (1986) he describes his recovery following a major injury to his left leg. Not only did the doctor become (temporarily at least) the patient, but in what he describes as 'a neurological novel', many themes he writes of touch on the experiences of recovering from a subarachnoid haemorrhage, including 'the business of being a patient and of returning later to the outside world' (1986: viii). Jane Grant, who had a below-the-knee amputation following a road accident, describes how from early on in her hospital stay she felt compelled to read others' narratives of trauma, illness and recovery (Grant 2006). In a sense, this is what I am perhaps doing here.

I have also cited from the research literature relating to outcomes and recovery from subarachnoid haemorrhage (Chapter 2). These research findings and conclusions are included to juxtapose, where relevant, these 'professional' perspectives with those whose lives have been directly affected. Presenting these 'parallel narratives' gives a voice to survivors of brain haemorrhage and to researchers/

clinicians. Writing from the perspective of a clinical practitioner who also writes 'neurological tales [describing] ordinary people', Paul Broks suggests that 'sometimes you are talking about the brain and sometimes about the person, the self' (2003: 130). He continues:

> One has to be bilingual, switching from the language of neuroscience to the language of experience; from talk of 'brain systems' and 'pathology', to talk of 'hope', 'dread', 'pain', 'joy', 'loss', 'love' . . .
>
> (Broks 2003: 130)

This chapter closes with an outline of the contents of this book.

What this book is about

Part I sets the scene, with four chapters, starting with this background chapter. Chapter 2 is an introduction to subarachnoid haemorrhage. It opens with a variety of definitions and descriptions, ranging from survivors' own descriptions, through to clinical and research perspectives and continues with an overview of: incidence, causes, risk factors, diagnosis and treatment, survival rates and outcomes. The chapter concludes with an overview of recent research studies into psychosocial outcomes of subarachnoid haemorrhage.

Chapter 3 introduces the people who were interviewed or who provided written accounts. It describes: recruitment methods; criteria for inclusion; survivors' reasons for agreeing to be interviewed and my methodology. Finally, there is a discussion about people writing about their recovery from brain haemorrhage. Chapter 4 discusses some broad themes of recovery: the individual nature of recovery; timescales of recovery; the non-linear nature of recovery; factors which may affect recovery; and subarachnoid haemorrhage as a 'hidden' disability. The chapter concludes with a discussion of trauma and recovery.

Part II discusses some specific aspects of recovery. Chapter 5 describes people's experiences of leaving specialist neurosurgical care, sometimes being transferred to a general hospital, before then returning home. Experiences of this early stage of recovery can be mixed, including relief at having survived a life-threatening event alongside feelings of loss of the safety or security of 'neurocare'. Memories of their hospital stay can be patchy so people may try to recover this 'lost time' and capture a fuller understanding of what they have been through.

Chapter 6 reports on people's experiences of information, advice and support services which they were offered before leaving hospital or shortly afterwards, and the kind of support they would like to have been able to access. The chapter goes on to discuss experiences of using community-based and outpatient services including specialist nurses, support groups and GPs. It also describes how people used the internet for information and advice, but also as a source of support through message boards and discussion groups.

Chapter 7 focuses on physical and sensory difficulties, including general physical mobility, eyesight, epilepsy, fatigue, sleep disturbance, headaches and head pain, taste and smell, unusual sensations and changes to physical appearance. All these difficulties have implications for survivors' psychosocial recovery.

Chapter 8 explores some of the ways in which a brain haemorrhage can affect people's cognitive functioning and abilities such as concentration, short-term memory, language, etc. As with physical difficulties, cognitive effects, however subtle, can have a significant effect on people's day-to-day life, though they were sometimes able to lessen their impact by finding ways of performing tasks differently.

The emotional impact of subarachnoid haemorrhage is the subject of Chapter 9. People describe how the haemorrhage generally affected the way they felt and the chapter continues with a discussion of more specific after-effects including anxiety, depression, loss of self-confidence and self-esteem, coping with enforced dependency and loss of autonomy, anger and frustration, and self-blame.

Part III turns to people's 'outer world' – their families and friends and the implications for their future employment. Chapter 10 describes how people's relationships with family members were affected by the haemorrhage, focusing on couples, their children and families in general. The chapter then discusses the role of friends in recovery: their initial reactions, their understanding of the haemorrhage and the part they played in helping people to recover. People's usual patterns of leisure and social activities are commonly affected – either in the immediate aftermath or in the longer term – and this is the subject of Chapter 11. The chapter discusses how the haemorrhage affected their social life, going out, driving, and home-based leisure activities, including reading and watching television.

Many people will have been in paid employment at the time of their haemorrhage and this is the subject of Chapter 12. It describes people's concerns about returning to work, deciding whether to return to their former job (if this was possible), how the return was negotiated with employers and their experiences of going back to work. Others describe how resuming former employment has not been possible and the development of alternatives, including retraining, career change and voluntary work. The chapter concludes with a discussion of the financial impact of unemployment following a haemorrhage.

The book closes with Part IV, 'Making Sense of It All'. Chapter 13 describes the varied 'tools for recovery' which individuals found had helped them to recover. Their suggestions cover areas as wide-ranging as their overall approach to recovery, setting goals and marking their achievements, acceptance and adjustment, self-compassion, physical self-care, the use of humour and finding help from books.

The final chapter, Chapter 14, brings together people's reflections on how the haemorrhage has changed their lives. They describe not only how their outlook on life has changed but also their sometimes altered view of themselves – the 'changed self'. The remaining sections discuss whether people felt they had been 'lucky' to survive, what they saw as the gains and losses of the experience and whether they felt they had 'got back to normal'.

Appendix A has brief details of the 27 people interviewed for this book and three people who wrote about their experiences in response to a questionnaire based on the topic guide used for interviews. Appendix B lists organisations and websites which can provide information and advice. Appendix C lists the support groups which were running at the end of 2007, together with their contact details. Appendix D is a glossary of terms.

2

SUBARACHNOID HAEMORRHAGE

An introduction

Definitions and descriptions

Subarachnoid haemorrhage is 'a leakage of blood that occurs over the surface of the brain, most commonly originating from a weakened artery deep within the brain' (Foulkes 2004: 5). This weakened artery can then form 'a balloon-like swelling called an aneurysm [and] the haemorrhage occurs when the aneurysm wall tears because of the pressure of blood' (Brain and Spine Foundation 2002: 4). Because aneurysms often resemble small red berries (or balloons) they are also sometimes referred to as 'berry aneurysms'. More detailed medical information can be found elsewhere (e.g. Lindsay and Bone 1997; Brain and Spine Foundation 2002; Foulkes 2004).

A haemorrhage frequently occurs without any warning and is potentially life threatening; it is described variously as an 'acute life-threatening illness . . . [and] a major life event' (Pritchard et al. 2001: 456, 461); and as a 'potentially lethal event [and] a medical emergency' (Vega et al. 2002: 601). These are how researchers and clinicians describe it, but when someone has had a haemorrhage, how do they define the experience? Survivors also had their own ways of describing what had happened to them.

When I asked the survivors, their responses varied. For Andrew, it was about 'serious illness, if you like to call it that, or a very serious experience'. Karen talked of how she 'looks upon it as an illness', but continued: 'You know it's not really an injury to me, it's not really an injury . . . [but] illness isn't quite right, is it? But it's still ongoing . . . if I'm not well, what do I call it?' Sandra and Roy both described it as an 'episode' or an 'event', and Pam and Vernon referred to it is an 'accident'. In Wendy's case, perhaps because of her nursing background, she explained how 'if I'm talking to someone medical, then I'll say "it was a subarachnoid"'. Maybe these are all ways of people trying to understand what had happened to them – or how to explain this to others. Thinking about their recovery, perhaps they aren't always sure whether or not they are ill, or indeed whether they are recovering from an illness. Sometimes people used images instead; Lauren talked of how

> the jigsaw had been thrown up into the air and pieces were scattered . . . and another picture I had in my head was that of a library where all the bookshelves had been overturned, all the books scattered all over.

Andrew reflected on what had happened:

> I looked and thought, my life is like a pack of cards and I felt I had a nice orderly pack, all just so! And they'd suddenly been shuffled and thrown all over the place – and I'm picking them up – I'm still picking them up to some extent and that's how it goes.

Whether it was a jigsaw where the pieces need to be fitted together (so that a complete picture emerged?), a library where not only the books but the shelves too had been overturned, or a randomly scattered pack of cards – all these images vividly convey a sudden event leaving a scene in disarray and disorder – and a consequent need to sort out, piece together, re-view and re-order. So these are not only images of brain haemorrhage but also images of recovery.

Survivors sometimes described their experiences of recovery in mechanistic terms; the brain is a machine, but now the machinery isn't working too well. For Janice, with her recovering brain it felt like 'the switchboard lights are all coming back on . . . it's all starting to work again'. Lesley described how, initially at least, she could only think very very slowly – 'as if my brain was a machine that had seized up . . . it was just taking an inordinately long time for the cogs to start moving and even then, they were a bit kind of graunchy' (i.e. making a crunching or a grinding sound). Wendy recalled her husband's description of her tired brain being 'like a rechargeable battery . . . when it's all charged up, if you've had a good sleep, you can do all those things, but if you do too much, too quickly, or you just don't stop, then you just grind to a halt'.

Some readers may want more factual information, which is the next section of this chapter.

Facts and figures about subarachnoid haemorrhage

Causes

Seventy-five per cent of haemorrhages are due to a ruptured aneurysm, 20 per cent have no identifiable cause and no aneurysm will be detected, and 5 per cent are caused by rare disorders including arteriovenous malformation (AVM) (Al-Shahi et al. 2006).

Incidence

Each year, between 10 and 15 people per 100,000 will be affected (Lindsay and Bone 1997; Foulkes 2004), the rates varying from country to country. More recently, however, it has been suggested that the incidence is about 8 per 100,000, leading to about 20 admissions a year to a general hospital (Al-Shahi et al. 2006). According to the Brain and Spine Foundation (2002), annually 8500 people in the UK will be affected.

Age

Subarachnoid haemorrhage becomes more common as people grow older (Brain and Spine Foundation 2002; Nursing Times 2005), but although the incidence increases with age, half will be under 55 years old at the time (van Gjin et al. 2007).

Gender

The incidence is roughly the same for men and women up to the age of 45, but then becomes more common amongst women (Pobereskin 2001). Across all age groups, two out of every three subarachnoid haemorrhages occur in women.

Risk factors

Our understanding of why aneurysms develop in the brain and why some of these subsequently rupture is incomplete, but it has been established that people who smoke or who have high blood pressure (hypertension), or who use alcohol excessively are at an increased risk for subarachnoid haemorrhage (Al-Shahi *et al.* 2006; van Gjin *et al.* 2007). It has also been suggested that abuse of recreational drugs may be associated with neurological syndromes, including subarachnoid haemorrhage (Enevoldson 2004). Genetic factors also account for one out of every ten subarachnoid haemorrhages (van Gjin *et al.* 2007) However, a haemorrhage can also occur to people where none of these risk factors are present (Brain and Spine Foundation 2002).

Diagnosis and treatment

The haemorrhage is usually diagnosed by a CT scan and/or lumbar puncture. A cerebral angiogram may also be performed to ascertain the cause of the haemorrhage. The ruptured aneurysm is usually treated either by clipping or by coiling. With clipping, a small metal or plastic clip is placed across the neck of the aneurysm to seal it off. With coiling (also described as embolisation), platinum coils or spirals are introduced into the aneurysm until blood can no longer enter it. Coiling is increasingly common these days, although it is not always possible, in which case the aneurysm is clipped. (These procedures are explained in more detail in patient and carer information booklets, e.g. Foulkes 2004; Brain and Spine Foundation 2002, 2005a.)

It may be of interest to see how treatments have moved on since 1931 when the *Canadian Medical Association Journal* reported on 'A Case of Subarachnoid Haemorrhage with Recovery'. After diagnosing this 35-year-old man by lumbar puncture, his doctors concluded: 'Treatment of this condition is simple. It consists in early and repeated lumbar punctures . . . he should be isolated and kept as quiet and comfortable as possible, with the milder sedatives. Enemata should be avoided' (Hutchinson and Baillie 1932: 509–12).

Survival rates

About 30 per cent of people who have a subarachnoid haemorrhage die within 24 hours and a further 25–30 per cent within four weeks (NICE 2005), but early diagnosis and treatment can improve the outcome and there has been a slight reduction in overall mortality rates between 1960 and the mid-1990s (Al-Shahi *et al.* 2006) and a trend towards gradual improvement (van Gjin *et al.* 2007).

Outcomes of subarachnoid haemorrhage

Although there has been this modest improvement in survival rates, as researchers (e.g. Beristain *et al.* 1996) have pointed out, further investigation of the quality of life and psychosocial outcomes is needed for those who do survive. Two important findings are emerging: first, that survivors, their relatives and neurosurgeons may have rather different views about what constitutes a 'good recovery'; second, outcomes must be viewed from a more holistic perspective which considers the survivor's overall quality of life.

Differing perspectives

Until researchers began to look more closely at the psychological and social effects of subarachnoid haemorrhage, the outcomes were generally measured in terms of someone's neurological recovery, using the Glasgow Outcome Scale (GOS). A 'good outcome', according to GOS, indicates that a person will be independent in daily life. However, an assessment that someone has made a 'good recovery' may result in an incomplete picture. This may be because:

> Neurosurgeons know all too well that SAH can kill or profoundly disable . . . [so] they may have a tendency to assess outcome by comparing it with 'what could have been'. However, patients and relatives, may be more likely to assess outcome by comparing it with 'what was'.
>
> (Buchanan *et al.* 2000: 836)

It was this perspective on recovery that led Buchanan *et al.* to ask patients and their relatives about how they viewed the outcomes after surgery and looked at these alongside the neurosurgeons' classification. After presenting their findings, they concluded: 'There are many facets to outcome and the patient, the relative and the neurosurgeon may view them differently. "Good" recovery is in the eye of the beholder' (Buchanan *et al.* 2000: 837).

Outcomes and quality of life

Over the last few years, several researchers (e.g. Hütter *et al.* 1995; Beristain *et al.* 1996; Ogden *et al.* 1997; Buchanan *et al.* 2000; Jarvis 2002) have drawn attention to the limitations of neurological measures, such as the GOS, which are insufficient to assess all the relevant aspects of quality of life (Hütter *et al.* 1995). We need 'a more complete vision of what it is that constitutes a good recovery' (Jarvis 2002: 1431). 'The concept of "outcome" in neurosurgery needs to be revised and updated' (Beristain *et al.* 1996: 422) to include survivors' subjective feelings of physical, psychological and social well-being.

Studies of psychosocial outcomes

A number of studies have now been completed which focus on psychosocial outcomes and offer a broader view of how subarachnoid haemorrhage can affect the survivor's quality of life. Although these are cited in various other chapters, the main findings from two recent UK studies are set out below.

Pritchard and his colleagues (2001) explored the psychosocial outcomes for 137 adults and their carers, who had been treated at a regional neurological centre. Although these survivors were generally very satisfied with their inpatient care, nearly half had experienced significant psychosocial difficulties after they returned home, including depression, anxiety, isolation and pain. Facing quite lengthy periods of being unable to work also had economic and social costs There was considerable dissatisfaction with advice and support, particularly when someone was seeking help with specific issues. This study contributed significantly to consumer-led research; participants were asked specific questions, but open-ended questions also enabled them to describe their experiences more fully. A very positive 'outcome' that emerged from this study was the health authority's decision to appoint a specialist liaison nurse service which also includes the provision of a support group (see Chapter 6 and Appendix C).

Another major study (Powell *et al.* 2002, 2004) also focused on psychosocial outcomes, involving 52 people considered to have made a 'good neurological recovery from aneurysmal SAH'. This study investigated the prevalence of psychosocial and cognitive difficulties, including post-traumatic stress symptoms; and also explored pre-illness stress and the relationship between emotional and functional outcomes. Participants in this study were interviewed at three, nine and 18 months post-discharge and completed a series of questionnaires and tests.

At nine months, the researchers found that a substantial proportion of these patients had 'protracted disturbances of mood, particularly with symptoms characteristic of post-traumatic stress, increased dependence on others for help with domestic and organisational activities, and reduced levels of productive employment' (Powell *et al.* 2002: 780). At 18 months, the majority of participants had no marked cognitive impairments or physical disability, but almost half were still dependent on others for help with daily living activities and had low levels of productive employment. Although this suggested that these patterns may have become entrenched or established since the haemorrhage, the researchers also pointed out that this may be – as some survivors had observed – that it 'had prompted them to re-appraise their lifestyle and adjust their lifestyles accordingly' (Powell *et al.* 2004: 1123). People's mood states had improved, but anxiety and depression were, respectively, three times and twice as high as those reported by healthy controls (Powell *et al.* 2004).

Both these studies contribute to our understanding of the psychosocial issues facing people recovering from subarachnoid haemorrhage, but equally importantly both drew attention to the need for more structured interventions post-discharge to address people's continuing difficulties:

> Appropriate clinical interventions must depend not only on what has changed, but on an understanding of the immediate and secondary psychological reactions that individual patients experience to their illness, hospitalisation and subsequent symptomatology. Where patients' horizons become limited by health anxieties, fatigue or a loss of confidence in their abilities, support and information from a knowledgeable professional after hospital discharge may be sufficient to dispel inaccurate beliefs and prevent avoidable problems developing. In other cases, it may be appropriate to provide access to more specialist interventions – for instance from a psychologist or an occupational therapist – to overcome potentially debilitating mood disturbances or directly assist the patient to re-engage with activities of daily living and regaining their personal autonomy.
>
> (Powell *et al.* 2004: 1124)

These and other studies have helped to increase our awareness of the outcomes and the kinds of difficulties which survivors may face during their recovery.

3

PERSONAL EXPERIENCES OF SUBARACHNOID HAEMORRHAGE

This chapter introduces the 27 people I interviewed for this book and a further three people who contributed written accounts. Factual information about these 30 people can be found in Appendix A. With their agreement, I have used participants' first names (except in cases where more than one person shared the same first names so these, with their agreement, were changed).

Recruiting survivors

I recruited survivors from the following sources.

- The Brain and Spine Foundation: information about the book was posted on their moderated discussion forum and a background information sheet was also sent to participants in a questionnaire survey the foundation was undertaking (see C.R. Scott 2006).
- Wessex and Greater Manchester Neuroscience Centres: Information was posted on the discussion board of their subarachnoid haemorrhage website. Although the discussion board has since closed down, the website with information about subarachnoid haemorrhage continues (see Appendix B).
- Wessex Neurological Centre: information was circulated by the specialist nurses and within their subarachnoid haemorrhage support group.
- British Association for Counselling and Psychotherapy: a notice was placed in the BACP journal, *Therapy Today*.
- Val Hennessy Trust, Coventry.
- Personal contacts; snowballing.

People who expressed an interest in being interviewed were sent some background information about the proposed book, its aims and intended readership. It also listed the following criteria for being interviewed which were that:

- the haemorrhage had occurred at least six months ago
- they had made – or were making – a 'good recovery' or were 'moderately disabled' (see below)
- they were able to undertake an interview of about one and a half to two hours (excluding breaks).

There were two reasons why I decided to exclude anyone whose haemorrhage had occurred within the previous six months. First, they may not have recovered to the point where they could undertake what would be a fairly lengthy interview. Second, insufficient time would possibly have elapsed for people to be able to gain some perspectives on their experiences of recovery.

The second criterion was loosely based on Scores 4 and 5 of the Glasgow Outcome Scale (see e.g. Powell *et al.* 2004):

- 5 = good recovery: able to resume normal activities although there may be minor neurological or psychological deficits
- 4 = moderately disabled: independent and can resume almost all activities of daily living; disabled to the extent that they cannot participate in a variety of social and work activities; disabilities include varying degrees of dysphasia, hemiparesis or ataxia as well as intellectual and memory deficits and personality changes.

Although participants did not necessarily know their GOS and were not asked to provide any clinical information about themselves, the terms 'good recovery' and 'moderately disabled' were used to ensure, as far as possible, that they would be able to be interviewed. When someone decided they would like to be interviewed, they received an information sheet about how, where and when the interviews would take place. They were also asked to sign a consent form.

The survivors

Information was obtained from 30 people (including three written accounts) and of these:

- 70 per cent were female and 30 per cent male. This broadly reflects the differing incidences for men and women (see p. 35) and the gender ratio is similar to the participants in two major studies of psychosocial outcomes (Pritchard *et al.* 2001; Powell *et al.* 2002, 2004)
- the youngest person was 23 at the time of their haemorrhage and the oldest was 68 (and in full-time employment)
- the average age was just over 45 years
- three people were in their twenties, three in their thirties, 13 in their forties, ten in their fifties and one in his sixties;
- 25 people had had a haemorrhage within the last five years.

Clinical data, such as the size and location of the aneurysm(s), were not routinely requested, but the following provides some information, based on what people had understood about their haemorrhage and how they explained this during the interview:

- In the vast majority of cases, the haemorrhage was caused by a ruptured aneurysm.
- In a very small number of cases, no aneurysm was found, although there had been a subarachnoid haemorrhage.
- One person's haemorrhage was caused by arteriovenous mal-formation (AVM) – an abnormality present from birth.
- One person had had a perimesencephalic haemorrhage – a variant of subarachnoid haemorrhage, where there is no aneurysm (Hop *et al.* 1998).
- Several people were found to have more than one aneurysm.
- Three people had had more than one haemorrhage.
- A small number of people had had a haemorrhagic stroke.

Despite these individual variations, as the following chapters illustrate, there are many shared features in people's experiences of recovery.

The interviews

The topic guide

I carried out the interviews using a semi-structured topic guide which, with one or two changes, was broadly based on HSQuale, an instrument for measuring the quality of life of young haemor-rhagic stroke victims (Hamedani *et al.* 2001). It had recently been used for a quality-of-life study of coping skills after subarachnoid haemorrhage (C.R. Scott 2006) which suggested that it would be appropriate. My topic guide covered ten main areas:

- the onset of the haemorrhage and hospital stay
- information, advice and support services after leaving hospital
- physical functioning
- cognitive functioning
- emotional well-being
- relationships with others
- social life and leisure activities
- employment
- coping strategies for recovery
- subarachnoid haemorrhage as a life-changing event.

Although the topic guide could have seemed rather dry or clinical, I saw the interviews as offering people the opportunity to recount their stories and to be able to reflect on their journeys of recovery, of how they had 'lived to tell the tale'. As narrative researcher Kim Etherington suggests:

> When people tell us their stories, we hear their feelings, thoughts and attitudes, and the richness of the narratives helps us to understand how they understand themselves, their strategies for coping and how they make theoretical sense of their lives.
>
> (Etherington 2002: 167)

The content of the interviews

Although not included in the HSQuale instrument, I decided to start the interviews by asking people to describe for me what had happened when the haemorrhage occurred and their subsequent hospital admission. This runs somewhat counter to the advice that qualitative research interviews should start with an open-ended non-threatening question (DiCiccio-Bloom and Crabtree 2006). Starting the interview by asking people to talk about such a traumatic event might have been risky or considered 'bad practice'. However, because participants were aware that I had been through a broadly similar experience, this perhaps made it easier, even though they were talking to a comparative stranger.

Before the recording started I did, in fact, have a preliminary question to test the recording equipment. I asked people to tell me what they'd had for supper the previous evening. In the event this wasn't always as unthreatening as I'd hoped it would be. Short-term memory problems sometimes left people struggling for an answer but it did act as an unintentional ice-breaker!

This semi-structured approach meant that other themes could emerge during the interviews (DiCiccio-Bloom and Crabtree 2006): for example, anxieties about resuming sexual activity post-haemorrhage (see pp. 159–60); the impact of the haemorrhage on the family's financial situation (see pp. 197–8); I also added two further questions after the first few interviews: the impact of the haemorrhage on their self-confidence; and how they had reacted to the potential loss of control implicit in the sudden onset of the haemorrhage. Having less structure can be more empowering for the person being interviewed (Wallcraft 2002) and enables them to frame their experiences in their own words. On the other hand, having some structure was also important in helping people keep 'on track'. Because of cognitive difficulties, there were times when people would start to talk about something, but then lose track of what they were saying and be unable to remember the question.

Setting up the interviews

The majority of interviews took place from mid-morning to late afternoon. There was a particular reason for this; a significant number of survivors were still grappling with mental fatigue (see pp. 108–11). Two people were interviewed in the evening because both had resumed full-time employment. Although family carers were not interviewed, two people asked if their spouse could also be present during the interview. This was mainly because they were concerned that their memory might be unreliable and they might need an occasional prompt.

Doing the interviews

I carried out the interviews between May and October 2006. The average length of interviews was between one and a half and two hours, the shortest being just under an hour, and the longest about two and a half hours. The information I sent out before the interviews included a brief statement that I had had a subarachnoid haemorrhage in 2001. As a result, people sometimes wanted to hear about my experiences of recovery. While this inevitably lengthened the interview, it also meant that there was a two-way process and at times the interviewer could share information and experiences which may have been helpful to the interviewee.

Because the interviews frequently developed a rather conversational style as experiences were shared by both parties, perhaps this enabled people to feel more comfortable with recounting events which might have evoked some strong feelings due to the traumatic nature of what had happened to them.

Analysing the interviews

The interviews were tape-recorded and transcribed word for word. I analysed the material using deductive or thematic analysis (Ely *et al.* 1997), based on the main themes in the topic guide, but also allowing for new themes to emerge in the course of the interviews.

Survivors' reasons for being interviewed

By agreeing to be interviewed, it was reasonable to assume that survivors were willing to talk about their experiences, but at the conclusion of each interview I asked what their reasons were for participating. By asking this at the end, they might also be clearer about how they had experienced the interview. The responses suggest that there are two main reasons – a wish to help others but also to benefit themselves in some way. As Andrew explained: 'It's always great to use what appears to be a bad experience, turn it around and get something positive out of it, because I think not only do other people benefit, but I think you benefit as well.'

Many people expressed the hope that by contributing to the book this would benefit others in a number of different ways. They wanted people to be able to access more comprehensive information, to give them hope for the future, to help them come to terms with what had happened and, by normalising people's experiences, to help them to feel less isolated:

I think it's good to be able to also read people's experiences because sometimes you just feel like a lunatic with what you've experienced. You don't know whether it's quite normal to feel the way that you do and I think it's really quite reassuring to know that other people have experienced [something] similar, or can even be worse than you are.

(Karen)

I feel it's a very helpful thing . . . I had nowhere to turn at all after mine. Just reading people's experiences or listening to people's experiences helps you, because you just think – there's light at the end of the tunnel.

(Patsy)

If your book will help other people come to terms with what's happened, it's a good thing!

(Jan)

I want to give people hope. The fact is that it's not all doom and gloom when you've had a brain haemorrhage. You can lead an almost normal life.

(Roy)

When I had [the haemorrhage], I thought I was the only person that had ever had it. I couldn't put the 2 per cent of the population into context. And when you said . . . that you were going to write this . . . I thought to myself, somebody in the same position as me [that] had nothing, this book would be marvellous, to see it from different people's points of view so that at least you can say 'that sounds similar to me' . . . so it's a realistic look at recovery – and hope.

(Karen-Ann)

The need to raise awareness about brain haemorrhages and recovery was also mentioned, which may lead to improved support services after people leave hospital:

Anything that can raise awareness as to the problem, which can happen to anyone, I will do my bit.

(Graham)

There's so little understanding out there around brain injury, [about] subarachnoid and because people don't realise the huge effort it takes to recover [and] that there need to be more support services in place.

(Lauren)

Wanting to help other people was not the only reason why people decided to be interviewed. Those who felt that they had ultimately gained from the experience, wanted to share this with others:

Why did I offer? . . . I think if it's going to help anyone, then I'm prepared to give whatever I can . . . it's a case that you want to give back, because I've reaped the benefit of different things.

(Veronica)

I feel it's been a positive experience for me, and I'm happy to share it, and it feels like part of that opportunity . . . It almost feels incumbent on me to make use of what I learned, that would be a rejection of what I've gone through.

(Lesley)

Being interviewed or providing a written account of their recovery had also offered people the chance to stand back and reflect on what had been happening:

That's almost like I've reached a point of being able to analyse things. Looking back on it I've been able to analyse it and work out more sort of whys and whats . . . I don't know whether I've actually sort of thought it through really before, talked it through.

(Christine)

I had been meaning for some time to write down my experiences to nail down the feelings and conclusions – this provided the spur for that.

(John)

Although most people who were interviewed were well on the road to recovery, they were still keen to read about other survivors' experiences:

47

It's going be really interesting to look at the book and see all the different experiences and how different they are . . . They're all like a story to be told.

(Vernon)

The book will be fascinating for me to read; to read about other people's experiences and to see how they've dealt with the problems which, obviously, lots of us are going through. And it's just great to meet you as well because you've been through it as well.

(Heather)

Although Faith's haemorrhage was over 20 years ago, she decided to be interviewed because she was 'very curious' having never been aware that recovery 'was a kind of topic in its own right'. The day after the interview, she wrote: 'It was a strange experience to dig up and examine long-buried memories. Quite cathartic.' Faith's experience of catharsis may have touched on something more widely shared. Reflecting on why she'd agreed to be interviewed Tania said: 'I think everyone's feeling a compulsion to tell their story, you know, me as well. And I think I talk too much about it sometimes . . . It's just getting over it, you can't stop talking about it.' Recounting the experience can enable the survivor to integrate the experience into their life story (Herman 1994).

Written accounts

It is becoming increasingly common for people to write about their experiences of illness and disability, whether as blogs posted on the internet, as books, magazine and newspaper articles, or as journals written for the writer's eyes only. Personal accounts can be found on the websites of most of the organisations listed in Appendix B. Although I didn't ask people whether they had written anything about their experiences of the haemorrhage and recovery, several offered to show me notebooks or diaries they had written and some had returned to reading these before the interview.

Personal accounts of illness or injury may be produced for several different reasons, not least because our life story, our personal narrative, is changed by these events. Writing can be an attempt to control the uncontrollable and contain the uncontainable, to put it outside one's self, and to try and make sense of what has happened. The words may even act as an 'anchor in turbulent seas' (Rimmon-Kenan 2005). Perhaps after a brain haemorrhage it could be important to prove to yourself – or others – that you could still string words together which made some sense. Writing about a traumatic event may also be beneficial, resulting in more positive moods and improvements to the immune system (Pennebaker et al. 1988).

Personal narratives are just that – personal and unique to that person. As Vernon pointed out, 'people's experiences are all totally different in their own way; they're all like a story to be told'. Research into the outcomes of brain haemorrhage can present glimpses of individual stories (e.g. Pritchard et al. 2001) by quoting directly from interviews with patients and carers. A study of personal accounts of illness on the internet pointed out that 'people are given a space to articulate their experiences, perceptions and understandings [and] such accounts provide insights into how bodily and emotional changes related to sickness are understood outside the prevailing bio-medical model' (Hardey 2002: 31). The details of individual stories paint a wider picture – a complex mix of events, ideas and experiences.

For some people, writing was a way of remembering the story. Veronica, who kept a diary in hospital and continued this for some time after she went home, is pleased to have this record because 'otherwise I would have forgotten [because] you do forget. Rereading it before the interview, she realised there were things she wanted to say but had forgotten.

Rather than having a diary or other written record to serve as a reminder, others may have written down the event in order to put it behind them and move on. Janice wrote about her experiences to be able to close that chapter of her life: 'I used to write an awful lot of stuff down in the early days. I've always done that, I've always written down how I feel about things . . . by writing it down then I can close the book.' Perhaps by doing this, it is also possible to get some sense of perspective about recent events? Andrew also wrote a great deal, perhaps in order to capture the learning or start to try and make sense of what had happened:

When I was home in the early days, I sat and wrote out lots of things. I wrote out what I thought were lots of truths about life, what the experience has shown me. At an early time I wrote down all the things that I felt I had learned through the experience.

Writing about the impact of your haemorrhage can also be a way of communicating to other people about what has happened – which sometimes isn't easy when they assume you have made a complete recovery. Shirley sent me several pieces of writing and in the first, entitled 'Normal', she explains:

> I find myself writing this down as it is the only way I think that people will understand . . . Because I look exactly as I did before, and I can talk properly and walk properly, everyone seems to think that everything is one hundred per cent. If I walked around with a bandage around my head, people could immediately see that I have a permanent injury.

Brian, whose employer already has inhouse blogs, decided to write 'The Positive Blog' after his haemorrhage – 'positive' because that was how he approached his recovery. He explains how both he and his colleagues have benefited from his decision:

> I'm looking at my recovery in a positive fashion and talking about it quite openly. Other people have read the blog and said 'you can't say this. It's very brave of you saying this in public!' Well no, this is how I really think. If it has helped one person who has a similar experience by them reading the blog and the phases I've gone through and where I've got help, etc., then that's fine . . . and there's a community in a large company and you don't realise there's a community, you think it's just people trying to do work, but I blogged about my injury and I got loads of responses.

Keeping some kind of diary, journal or written record can also provide useful evidence of progress during recovery, however, uneven that may be at times. As Wendy explained:

> I think for some people, keeping a diary can be quite useful because they can look back to what they were like when they

first came out of hospital, to what they're like a month later and sort of recognising that progress.

Andrew also recommended keeping some kind of written record of his progress:

> I kept odd notes about how I felt . . . the days that I felt really terrible, physically tired or emotionally sort of down . . . but I do think that it will be helpful to anyone, because you can look and you can see where you've made improvements . . . they can be very slow but when you look back over time you will see the improvements that are being made and I think it's important because it obviously helps you to reflect on what's going on . . . I found it useful for me.

Christine kept a written record for a while, partly so that she could be more specific about what was difficult on the bad days but also to try and understand whether there were particular reasons for her difficulties. Doing this has been a mixed experience:

> I went through a phase of keeping a little notebook because I kept thinking, well, when I feel good I forget about how bad I feel . . . I thought, well, I always find it difficult to say what actually specifically is wrong today, so I kept going for a little while . . . and then towards the end, I thought, I'm just obsessed with this but actually it's really interesting to look back on it now.

4

ASPECTS OF RECOVERY

'Recovery' or 'progress'?

This chapter explores some broader themes of recovery. More specific aspects of recovery are addressed in Parts II and III.

Although I am writing about 'recovery' and it forms part of the book's title, interestingly at least one person I interviewed questioned the use of that word. Sandra explained how she prefers to talk about 'progress – or whatever you like to call it'. Talking about progress suggests 'the action of stepping or moving forward or onward' (Shorter OED, Vol. II), whereas 'recovery' has the sense of going back or reclaiming something which has been lost. I continue to use the word recovery in this book, but Sandra's point seems worth including here.

Similar comments about the term 'recovery' were made by Sam, a 40-year-old man with traumatic brain injury who participated in a study by Nochi. 'Sam,' he writes, 'did not like to use a word like "recovery" because it was strongly associated with the pre-injury conditions . . . instead of that word, he concentrated on words like "progress" or "improvement" so that he could attach more significance to small, positive changes' (Nochi 2000: 1799).

Is recovery the same for everyone?

The ways in which people react, physically and psychologically, to surviving a brain haemorrhage, and their experiences in hospital and subsequent recovery will vary from person to person (Foulkes 2004; Powell *et al.* 2004). And recovery, it has been suggested, 'is a deeply personal, unique process of changing one's attitudes, values, feelings, goals, skills and/or roles. It is a way of living a satisfying, hopeful and contributing life despite the limitations caused by the illness' (Anthony 1993, cited in Wallcraft 2002).

Several people echoed this when talking about what they have found helpful during their recovery (see Chapter 13). As Christine said: 'There is no right or wrong way of dealing with anything . . . you just have to do what's right for you . . . we've had the same thing but completely different experiences and yet some bits are the same.' And Patsy concluded that 'we all deal with things differently . . . we all recover differently, don't we?'

Not only does the survivors' approach to their recovery vary, but as Scott found, other people's reactions can also vary: 'People's reaction to the haemorrhage is unpredictable. I know that no two haemorrhages are the same, but no two people's reaction to the haemorrhage is the same in terms of having it happen to somebody.'

Christine's point that there isn't a right or wrong way for people to approach their recovery sounds reassuring, but during some of the interviews it emerged that people wanted to find out how their recovery compared with others. There were spoken – or sometimes unspoken – questions: How am I doing? Am I doing well enough? Am I doing better or worse than other people who had a sub-arachnoid haemorrhage at the same time as me? This may be due to the fact that many individuals don't get to meet other people who are recovering – an issue we return to in Chapter 6.

If recovery is an individual journey or process, then the kinds of advice, information and support people receive after leaving hospital will need to be responsive to their individual circumstances. A one-size-fits-all response may not be sufficient: 'information materials were no substitute for case-specific help and advice' (Pritchard *et al.* 2001: 462).

What may affect recovery?

Survivors may want to know whether difficulties they are experiencing are caused by their brain injury. Is this necessarily the case? Do the size and site of the aneurysm and the severity of the bleed determine the extent of someone's post-haemorrhage difficulties? Or is recovery affected by this crisis in their health and the psychological effects of a traumatic and life-threatening event? As Jane Lapotaire's neuropsychologist explained to her:

> Dr Baehr just says, even more gently . . . you have a twofold crisis to manage. The emotional shock, the trauma

53

of being so near death and the physical side of being in intensive care that long, plus the insult to the brain that clipping an aneurysm causes.

(Lapotaire 2003: 259)

Studies of the psychosocial outcomes of subarachnoid haemorrhage suggest that there are different factors which interact with one other:

On the balance of the evidence, it seems probable that psychosocial problems following SAH are likely to reflect interactions between organic impairments, pre-existing life stressors, changes in social circumstances, or the occurrence of other stressors (such as reduced employment or lowered income) following the injury and non-specific reactions to life-threatening illness. While it is of theoretical interest to ascertain the extent to which problems are direct organic effects of the brain injury, these possible causal factors are so interconnected that the question is unlikely to be answerable with precision.

(Powell *et al.* 2002: 773)

Another study (Pritchard *et al.* 2001) found that people's age and gender, the time since their haemorrhage, and the size of bleed and site of the aneurysm did not relate specifically to their psychosocial difficulties afterwards. Perhaps, they suggested, these difficulties may have more to do with the way someone responds to a traumatic and life-threatening illness.

Even if age is not considered relevant to people's difficulties, nevertheless it was an issue for some of them. When asked by the interviewer whether they considered that their brain 'wasn't always working as well as it did before the haemorrhage', several people raised the issue of ageing. Lesley, who has short-term memory problems, replied: 'Memory – I would say, but I have to add the rider that I'm 55 so I can't say definitively that that's the case. It could be the ageing process.' With Andrew, even though he is only in his forties and his short-term memory has improved, this still worries him: 'Even to this day, I still have what you could say are "senior moments", I suppose and I'm never quite sure – it is still a hangover from the haemorrhage or is it just that . . . I'm getting on and people get like that?'

54

Fatigue, which is very common following a brain haemorrhage, also led Wendy to question whether this was age-related: 'I'm getting older, so is the tiredness I'm feeling [due to] my age? Or is it the fact that I had a brain haemorrhage four years ago? I'd like to blame it on the brain haemorrhage!' For Veronica, the life changes since her haemorrhage were inseparable from the changes which accompany ageing: 'Life does change; but then, I mean, I'm now 60 so I think your life does change as you get older, obviously.'

How long does it take to recover?

Wanting to find out how long her recovery would last, Tania recalls being given another question (rather than an answer): 'How long is a piece of string?' This was probably quite a good reply, but when they leave hospital most people will still want to know 'How long will it take me to get better?' And perhaps there's another question hovering around too: 'Can I expect to get back to normal?' People may want to be given a more or less definite timescale to recovery, but as Janice commented: 'With a brain injury, it's another thing really and you can't put a timescale on it. I think everybody's different; we're all individuals.' Health professionals advice would agree: 'Don't be concerned if your recovery period appears to differ from that of others, you will recover at your own pace' (Foulkes 2004). Another booklet suggests that 'it can take many months . . . to feel that life is getting back to "normal"' (Brain and Spine Foundation 2005b).

Nearly 20 years ago rather shorter timescales of recovery were envisaged, perhaps because there was less awareness of the psychosocial impact of subarachnoid haemorrhage, even when someone has made a good neurological recovery: 'The typical pattern in a straightforward case was a gentle convalescence and then the patient returning to a normal lifestyle by three months' (McKenna et al. 1989: 487). Faith, whose haemorrhage occurred just two years before that paper was published, reflects similar views about recovery (from both the doctor's and the patient's point of view). As she commented: 'Until I had [the haemorrhage] I took the view that illnesses were something that you had and then you recovered from and that was it, unless it was a terminal illness of course.' After leaving hospital, Faith spent some time in a convalescent home where the nurses told her how lucky she was so, as she said: 'You either had one and you were over it, and that was it, or else you'd be unlucky and die.'

People had been given a range of suggested timescales for recovery. Jessica was told 'several years' and Scott '18 months to three years'. Veronica was told 'a year or two years' and Pam 'about two years'. Karen-Ann's neurosurgeon was more cautious: 'It can take up to four years to see where you are and that wasn't necessarily for full recovery to get to be the person that you were before.' (Chapter 14 explores the theme of 'getting back to normal' more fully.)

It is understandable that people want some certainty, some idea of what their immediate future will be like and when and whether they will make a complete recovery, but as some people found, their recovery was going to take longer than expected. David began to realise how serious his haemorrhage had been:

> I knew then that it was going to be a lot longer slog than I had envisaged. I thought maybe a couple of months, but no, it's not been a couple of months . . . I'm well on the way to recovery, it's just a damn sight slower than I want it to be!

Although she was given no specific information about the expected length of recovery, Tania discovered for herself:

> Nobody talked about months and years . . . and in my head I was thinking about three months . . . you don't realise what a big deal the recovery is going to be and what's involved and how long it will take. I don't think they can really give you timescales, but they could have maybe said, think in terms of a few months and maybe wait until you're passed to drive again . . . because that could take six to ten months or so. [But] if someone had told me I'd be off work for just over two years, I would have been really shocked and upset . . . that must be difficult to take in and you'd wonder what on earth to fill your time with.

If recovery is frequently longer than people anticipated, they also found that problems could continue not just over months but over years. This is borne out by an Australian study of a group of people whose haemorrhage was between four and seven years ago. Many who had suffered from fatigue for months and years reported that they were now back to normal, suggesting that 'some symptoms typical of diffuse brain damage can continue to recover for many years' (Ogden et al. 1997: 32).

When Pam had a haemorrhagic stroke, she was told it would take about two years to recover fully. Although she thought at the time that this was realistic, she's also clear that her recovery does not have a finite point: 'I don't think I've recovered completely because something new happens every day, even if it might only be something little.' And Veronica, who'd been told recovery would possibly take a year or two found that 'this second year I've made as much of a recovery as I did the first year' and nearly three years down the road she feels she is still recovering. As Sandra described it: 'I think I'm in recovery, well, I hope for the rest of my life.'

Sometimes a complete recovery may not be possible, but when Claudia Osborn recognised that after her head injury there were some things she would never achieve, she still believes 'it is important that this ceiling idea not limit your recovery' (1998: 227). For Vernon, who acquired significant physical and cognitive disabilities following a haemorrhage eight years ago, his recovery has 'moved into something different'. Now he says: 'I'm not sure whether I need to rehabilitate any more, but I do need to look after myself as well at the same time . . . it's sort of like a continuum looking after yourself . . . somewhere along the line I've changed into that.'

One of the recurring themes in the interviews was that recovery can't be rushed. It has its own pace – its own timescales – and some survivors had learned to accept that. Lesley was told by her neurosurgeon that her recovery might take up to a year, but everyone is different and the timescale would depend on a number of factors. In fact it did take a year before she felt physically 'reasonably okay' but she found that adopting a more flexible approach worked better for her:

I'm not the sort of person who thinks, well . . . I should be better by such and such, or this is going to be all right by then. I just take things as they come . . . I'm also quite okay with allowing time to take its course. So it was just, okay, well, not right yet, but not really stressing about it at all and then just sort of celebrating when things felt better; that, I think, has always been my way really . . . maybe it's a bit laissez-faire but it seems to work for me.

For Christine too her recovery has had its own timescale. Seven years after her haemorrhage, she acknowledges that things can't be hurried along:

> I'm pretty sure that I will move on, because I've got through lots of stages . . . After twelve months I thought, oh, that's amazing, I feel great . . . and you realise actually – I wasn't anywhere near great at that point! So it's very very slow progress, very slow, but it *is* progress and you've just got to go through it.

Good days, bad days?

Several people compared the process of recovery to being on a journey: for Rosie 'it's a journey and it's exciting!'; for Lauren the 'whole trip has been very emotional but I've had to learn it as I've gone along really'. Although this suggests a journey that has been ultimately worthwhile, the route wasn't always smooth. 'There will be peaks and troughs, good days and bad. Don't give up hope during the bad days' is helpful advice from the Brain and Spine Foundation (2002: 16), but survivors may not realise this at first. As a nurse, Wendy already knew about anticipated pathways of recovery from surgery, so when she came out of hospital she assumed her recovery would follow a predictable sequence with clear phases:

> You know if you're having your appendix out, this is the plan of care that will happen to you and by such and such a time, you will be able to do this, that and the other. There isn't anything like that [for subarachnoid haemorrhage] so I didn't know whether what I was doing or how I was feeling were the same as everybody else; whether I was feeling better or . . . was I feeling much worse . . . I kept saying it's only a brain haemorrhage; I should be able to do this by now. If I'd broken my leg then I would know that it could take so many weeks, so many months, to get better.

When someone leaves hospital having been told they have made a good recovery, they may, not unreasonably, assume that their longer term recovery will continue uninterrupted. Veronica was told she had made 'an excellent recovery' and thought that progress would be continuous and uninterrupted so 'I expected it to carry on like that . . . at the time I didn't expect to go down again.' Even when she was told at her first outpatient appointment to expect ups and downs, she really didn't want to know: 'I needed positive information; I really didn't want any of the downside to it.'

Brian was eager to return to work as soon as possible, but discovered after he did so that recovery can have ups and downs – perhaps rather like a game of snakes and ladders – and progress wouldn't necessarily be even:

> I had a really good week and it went better and better and better. I was full of doing all the things that I do . . . The second week was just as good as I was getting better and better and better . . . the next week, on that Saturday I just felt so ill and so I'd gone up and up and up, and then just falling off this cliff! . . . I started feeling ill and I started getting more pains . . . Because I was feeling better, doing more and more and more, you want to push the envelope all the time, but you go too far, you fall off and you have a bad week – and I'd had a bad week! It's because I pushed myself too far . . . I want to get high up this recovery hill but I'm going to try and throttle back.

In the early stages of recovery, when the bad days are probably more likely to outnumber the good ones, Karen started keeping a count, but then realised this wasn't helpful:

> I was having a lot more bad days than good days, in fact I put it on the sheet over there. There was one month, I think I'd had three months of really bad times and then I had one day and I put it on the calendar that it was a really good day . . . next three months – absolute rubbish. I think it was from that point I thought I've just got to take everything one day at a time to be able to cope.

Four years after her haemorrhagic stroke, Pam still has bad days which are frustrating, though now she can see the broader picture – how much progress she has actually made during this time:

I'm really glad to have got this far because, looking at me when I came out of hospital . . . I'm a different person altogether. You wouldn't know it was the same person . . . But what is frustrating for me is some days I can write really well, like I did before, other days I just can't! I have to hold this hand with the [other] hand to keep it straight . . . some days it's very bad; other days it's fine which is frustrating . . . but there's no comparison with me now to when I came out of hospital.

'But you look normal!'

If someone leaves hospital with obvious physical difficulties – when they've had a stroke, for example – other people will be able to see that all is not well. When someone has been treated by coiling (see Glossary) there will be no visible signs. Even when the aneurysm has been clipped, the scar may be behind the hairline. But as Jane Lapotaire discovered:

Once the scar has healed and the hair regrown after a cerebral haemorrhage, the experience, as I continually discover, was at worst totally foreign to most people and at best misunderstood. The brain is left vulnerable to noise, physical jostling or any form of vocal and emotional harshness.
(Lapotaire 2003: xiii)

Several people, including Patsy, suggested that a bandage, or even a badge, would provide a visible signal:

If we had a bandage around our heads, people would say 'Are you okay?' . . . I was telling you about the lady who dropped something in the bank and I couldn't pick it up. Because I look okay everyone probably thought 'Oh why didn't she do that?' They don't understand. We ought to have a badge perhaps! But I suppose I was the same and didn't understand . . . until it happens to you.

Actually having a bandage can be welcome. After he returned home, Scott developed hydrocephalus and had to return to hospital for a shunt to be inserted. This time his injury was visible: 'I had a huge whacking bandage on my head and that was brilliant because finally people could see that there was something wrong with me.'

Finding a way to explain yourself to other people who declare you to be normal or who minimise your difficulties isn't easy:

> The ability to deal with other people's misconceptions and communicate openly and honestly is very challenging. What can the person with a brain injury say to the comment 'Oh, you do look well – there's nothing wrong with you', when they might have a number of hidden residual symptoms and feel awful. Or what can be said to the comment from others, 'I've got memory problems too' or 'I get tired too.'
>
> (Powell 2004: 193)

Wendy finds it difficult having to explain the effects of her haemorrhage to others: 'If I had a limp or something from it, then people would know that I've had something wrong with me and they might make excuses rather than me having to say to them "I'm like this because . . .".' Even when someone tries to explain to other people how the haemorrhage is affecting them, as Brian found, he wasn't always sure whether he'd got the message across:

> I don't know whether people understand. So every time friends came round to me, I would go on and on about, 'I'm having a good time with you now, but once you've left I shall go and lie down so I'm not really recovered.' I'll try and explain that again and again and you can never tell whether they've really got it.

Because recovery can last for months or even years, although someone may leave hospital with visible disabilities, once they have recovered physically to some extent then even people who know them may assume that recovery is complete. As Vernon found:

> I suppose if you or I had our legs or arms chopped off or something, people would kind of understand, but quite a few people have said 'Okay, you obviously didn't look normal when you came out of hospital but now you look perfectly normal' and I think people then just don't see some of the other bits.

Psychological scars are invisible and, as Andrew said: 'There's nothing to see on most people; maybe a scar, but they look at you and think, "Well, you look all right!" And yet they don't know what emotional baggage and stuff is going on inside . . . I might look all right but I don't actually feel emotionally right at all!'

Sometimes encountering people who know nothing about the haemorrhage can be difficult – not because they think you're okay but because they draw other conclusions. David's speech problems led to some misunderstandings on the part of people who knew him but hadn't heard about what had happened:

> If you have a broken leg, it's visible, they can see it's in plaster . . . with something to do with your brain, there's nothing there, so some people can be a bit naive and they'll think, well, what's wrong with him? Is he a drunk?

Perhaps this business of appearing 'normal' involves a two-way process – both parties want things to get back to normal as quickly as possible. Friends may, quite understandably, want things to return to how they were before, but the person who had the haemorrhage may also want to get back to their 'normal' pre-haemorrhage life as well. Veronica decided to return to college and continue the computer courses she'd previously been doing:

> because I felt I'd got to test my brain out . . . I found that very very difficult the first time back in college and sitting at the computer and reading these books and I had to really con-centrate hard . . . I just had to prove to myself and other people that my brain was still working.

When he returned to work, Roy also wanted to prove to his colleagues that he was able to do his job as well as before:

> I went back to work and it gave me the impetus to start saying – well, I'm back at work, I'm going to show them that I can do just as good a job as I did before I had [the haemorrhage] . . . I made a conscious effort of being aware of everything that I was supposed to do, everything that I was responsible for.

Recovery from trauma

Subarachnoid haemorrhage is a shocking event – 'a traumatic illness experience' (Jarvis 2002), 'a traumatic occurrence' (C.R. Scott 2006). Traumatic events occur suddenly and unexpectedly. As Joan Didion wrote of her husband's fatal heart attack: 'Life changes fast, life changes in an instant' (2006: 3). So how common is post-traumatic stress disorder (PTSD) after a brain haemorrhage when symptoms may include: intrusive memories of the traumatic event ('flashbacks'); avoiding reminders of the trauma; psychological numbness; and experiencing raised levels of arousal – being 'jumpy'. The results of several studies suggest that after subarachnoid haemorrhage survivors may experience some PTSD symptoms.

Pritchard *et al.* (2004: 25) identified what they describe as a 'global post-traumatic stress response [due to] acute cerebral damage [but also] a result of the nature of the event, not only the cerebral damage, but the sudden, catastrophic, life-threatening event in the lives of people, the majority of whom are at the peak of their family and professional responsibilities'. In many cases, post-traumatic stress reactions fade over time. Powell and his colleagues found that three months after the haemorrhage 60 per cent of people had at least one symptom of PTSD, but at nine months this had halved and at 18 months, although over 20 per cent still had frequent intrusive thoughts, only 6 per cent had clinically significant symptoms of intrusive thoughts and avoidance (Powell *et al.* 2002, 2004).

Another study (Sheldrick *et al.* 2006), investigating post-traumatic stress disorder in people who had suffered a subarachnoid haemorrhage or myocardial infarction, found that although symptoms of PTSD increased immediately after people left hospital, they subsequently lessened. Even though this may not be a long-term problem for most people, it does suggest that support and reassurance may be particularly important in the very early stages of recovery.

Although some survivors may have felt unwell for days or even weeks before being admitted to hospital, for many the haemorrhage came out of the blue with a sudden collapse. Megan was well aware of how abruptly life can change, even though on this occasion she'd survived:

I think what the brain haemorrhage has done is made me realise how life can change [snapping her fingers] just like that.

It can be a split second and everything can change . . . I was lucky this time [but] . . . I think it makes you realise the suddenness.

Since this sudden turn of events, Patsy finds she appreciates life more 'because we, more than anyone, know how quickly that all can change'.

Not only did the haemorrhage usually happen very suddenly, but this extraordinary event was in stark contrast to the very ordinary, unremarkable circumstances when people had collapsed:

Half an hour earlier I'd come back from work and the honey-suckle was growing over the window, as it does, and needed trimming back. So I was in the garden when I felt dizzy, like I was going to collapse and staggered into the kitchen, where I did collapse. I'd lost consciousness at that stage.

(Scott)

I'd just walked out of the house to work; it was about three minutes to twelve . . . and as I started to walk down the street I just collapsed; there was no pain or anything.

(Jessica)

I was sitting watching the television, like you usually do on a Saturday evening, chatting away to my partner, Mark . . . and halfway through the conversation I felt something pop.

(Karen-Ann)

I thought I'd better go and have some dinner. And as I was opening a tin of tuna, something happened in my head and I couldn't say what it was but . . . it felt like an explosion and I felt this pain, horrendous pain seemed to shoot down my whole body and it sort of knocked me to the floor. Then I had this incredible headache.

(Christine)

When someone is having a brain haemorrhage, they may lose con-sciousness or be semi-conscious, but still have intrusive memories of that time when they were critically ill. Fourteen years later, Kaz still has occasional flashbacks: 'I get a sudden flashback and I'll remember something like being wheeled down to theatre and my dad holding my hand, as I'm being wheeled down for my pre-med, and then I have to phone my parents and I say "Did this happen?"'

However, even when people were aware of what was happening, they sometimes reacted by battening down the emotional hatches – by being unnaturally calm perhaps – or by refusing to accept the diagnosis. When Wendy collapsed with a severe headache and vomiting, she thought that this was either a migraine attack or possibly meningitis: 'It didn't even cross my mind that it might be a haemorrhage.' After being transferred to a specialist neurology unit, she still found it hard to accept the diagnosis: 'I kept thinking, they've made a mistake because I wasn't paralysed. I kept thinking I've just got a headache, they must be wrong. There's an element of disbelief there, I think!'

Tania, on the other hand, did not question the diagnosis when told she was having a brain haemorrhage and her doctors explained about the aneurysm:

I listened, I understood, but I just didn't feel any kind of emotional impact. I knew I would need an operation, but I think I just couldn't take in the shock. I wasn't shocked, I was practical about it and just accepting that that [was] what I had to do.

Not allowing oneself to have any feelings about what is happening is often a natural way of protecting ourselves and managing a situation which might otherwise feel unmanageable. As Pam realised: 'I didn't feel, I wouldn't feel, it was too frightening to feel, so to cope I just didn't feel . . . so initially it was by denial and dissociation.' Only later, sometimes much later, does the reality of what has happened begin to sink in, an issue we return to in Chapter 5.

As Megan says 'everything can change'. Surviving a life-threatening event can challenge many of our 'basic assumptions' or beliefs about life and our place in it (Parkes 1998). After a brain haemorrhage, these more or less ordered patterns which give our life purpose and meaning are disrupted, for the time being at least:

People usually have assumptions of invulnerability, meaningfulness in life, personal control and positive self-regard.

These assumptions are challenged by traumatic events such as being diagnosed with a serious illness.

(Larner 2005: 37)

We generally assume that, apart from minor illnesses or injuries, our bodies are pretty invulnerable and reliable, but with brain haemorrhage that assumption will be overturned or at least come into question. For those who have had a haemorrhagic stroke, the body's very evident 'failure' will be particularly shocking:

I would brood on the paper-thin gap between health and sickness. As adults we forget that we live in our bodies. The unexpected failure of the body is a shocking catastrophe that threatens the flimsy edifice that we call the 'self'.

(McCrum 1998: 50)

When the haemorrhage occurs without warning, it brings us face to face with the fact that sometimes things happen which are beyond our control. Feeling we have some control over what happens to us helps us to feel self-confident, which in turn feeds into our self-esteem.

This has been a relatively brief discussion of the traumatic aspects of subarachnoid haemorrhage, but other possible reactions to trauma, notably anxiety, are discussed in Chapter 9. Chapter 14, the final chapter of this book, also looks at growing evidence that alongside suffering there can also be 'post-traumatic growth' (Linley and Joseph 2002).

Part II

RECOVERY

5

LEAVING HOSPITAL

Leaving the specialist unit

Just over half of survivors of subarachnoid haemorrhage go directly home from the specialist unit where they were treated. Almost a third will go to their local district general hospital for a few days to start their convalescence while the remainder, who need more specialist help and support at this stage, will spend time in a rehabilitation unit where they can receive services such as physiotherapy, speech and occupational therapy on an inpatient basis (Jarvis and Talbot 2004). Leaving neurocare can feel like a big step, so to understand the issues involved it is worth looking at how people felt about their time on the neurosurgical ward and what they were leaving behind when they were discharged.

Although by no means everyone will have clear memories of arriving at the neurosurgical unit, for some it had meant arriving at a place of safety. Whatever they had to go through subsequently, there was still this sense of being protected. Wendy arrived from her local hospital at the neurology department of a major teaching hospital and, as she recalls: 'It wasn't until I got there, I actually started to feel a bit safer.'

As Brian found, having a firm diagnosis and being told how his haemorrhage would be treated was a huge relief. As he says: 'At last! At last! Somebody's going to do something about it. And I wasn't scared; it's completely amazing.' The life-threatening nature of the event may only really sink in much later. Sandra reacted in a similar fashion, feeling that she could relinquish control and hand things over to the hospital staff:

> I was relieved that someone had actually recognised what it was, diagnosed it and they were dealing with it . . . I think it was

69

at that point that I started to relinquish all concerns and all anxieties and it was a case of, well, what's meant to be is meant to be . . . I'm being cared for now . . . Something kicked in that said, let it go . . . you're in their hands, there's absolutely nothing you can do.

Although the haemorrhage usually occurs suddenly, without warning, this isn't always the case. Karen had had similar though less severe symptoms four years ago, but test results at that time were inconclusive. When this time she collapsed and was admitted to a neurosurgical unit, she was thankful to have a clear diagnosis and treatment plan:

I thought after all those years from the first time it happened . . . something's going to happen and something's going to be fixed at long last and that was my main thing. I was just happy to be there and they were actually going to fix a problem and somebody believed me! . . . I was actually going to be taken care of.

The need for close observation and monitoring of patients means that there are high levels of care on a neurosurgical ward, providing what Kaz described as a 'security blanket'. These feelings of being cared for were commented on by several people like Christine: 'Fantastic. I can remember loving the gentleness, they were incredibly gentle and kind. It was the most kindness and gentleness and I remember thinking, these are such wonderful people, you know? They were really very good.' Wendy too appreciated the nursing on the high dependency unit where she spent the first few days:

There were nurses there all the time whenever you needed anything you know . . . you weren't allowed to move, you had to lay flat which is typical, but whenever you needed anything they were there. The nursing care was superb. I felt very safe in that environment.

The routine of the neurosurgical ward also had a reassuring quality. Despite the seriousness of the situation, Andrew said: 'It was strange because I felt a security being there and there was a regime; they would come in at set times and do set things.'

Being discharged after any time in hospital is often a cause for celebration, the next step on the journey of recovery, but as Veronica found there can be mixed feelings when the time comes:

When they told me I was coming home I was really really pleased . . . but I was terrified . . . and I was crying. I was really frightened about coming home because you feel quite sheltered whilst you are in hospital; everyone's there on hand.

Lesley Foulkes, a specialist nurse who runs the subarachnoid haemorrhage support group at Wessex Neurological Centre, sees how the hospital can come to represent a secure and known environment: 'For some people it's very safe; they feel safe coming back here and they feel it's familiar.' However, she also points out that this won't always be the case if the traumatic impact of the original hospital stay results in too many negative associations:

A few people have not been able to attend the support group because it's [coming] back to the unit – and not always the patients themselves but the family members find it's too anxiety provoking or too emotional to come back and they don't want to come back here. It's past, you know. It's a building that's all linked up with that horrific phase they they've moved on from.

On the way home: non-specialist hospital care

Depending on how quickly someone has recovered and how much support is available at home, survivors may be discharged back to the hospital from which they were originally admitted. Unfortunately, people's experiences of returning to non-specialist hospital care often compared unfavourably with their stay in a specialist unit. There are several possible reasons for this. Roy spent a week on what he described as a 'renal geriatrics' ward. This could have been an opportunity for staff to assess him for any services he might have needed but this is not what happened:

It was a nightmare! They had no real place for me at all; one surgeon came to see me and he said 'Hello, I'm Mr so-and-so' and I never saw him again. I never saw anybody. It was just a staging post. I stayed there for a week and then came home. I tried to get some physiotherapy and that was very very difficult to get hold of.

Lesley returned to the hospital which had referred her to the neurosurgical unit in another hospital, but communication between them seems to have broken down because:

They knew nothing about me, they said. I was a complete surprise to them! So as far as I was concerned, I was a body that [the neurosurgical unit] just needed to get rid of and they had to shove me somewhere at some point.

Janice's staging post, like some others, was a stroke unit, despite the fact that she hadn't had a stroke and as she recalls:

It was not a nice experience. I just said 'I'm fine. Let me go home – please, please, please.' I felt like I didn't exist. I was just . . . 'Let me get out of here!' I felt like I was in God's waiting room.

There is often likely to be pressure on bed spaces in neurosurgery units, but when existing patients are ready to be discharged inadequate liaison between specialist and general hospital care can result in problems with follow-up care. Scott described his experience of this as 'getting lost in the loop' which meant that some time elapsed before a proper package of care was organised for him at home.

Apart from any longer term arrangements when someone returns home, being moved on to a general ward could be a frightening experience when something goes astray. When Christine left neurocare she was still on the standard 21-day course of nimodipine (to prevent vasospasm), but the medication couldn't be found:

I remember they couldn't find the tablets I had because I remember saying, I hadn't had them, because I was so used to them. And every four hours I had these tablets and I hadn't had them and I remember actually saying 'I haven't had my [medication]' . . . and I could feel the panic . . . I was really scared.

Specialist liaison nurse, Anne Jarvis, proposes that a written document should accompany the patient when they transfer from the specialist unit to a district general hospital. If general hospital staff were also able to contact specialist nurses for further advice or information, they would then be able to offer patients appropriate and accurate information and advice about possible difficulties in recovery such as fatigue, cognitive problems and emotional changes (Jarvis 2002: 1436).

Residential rehabilitation units

A minority of survivors will spend some time in a rehabilitation centre, often because they have had a haemorrhagic stroke. Graham spent six months in a specialist residential centre which he describes as 'magnificent' where he was helped to read and write and walk again before he returned home. Jan also spent seven months in a rehabilitation centre where, despite continually demanding to be allowed to go home, she also found the staff 'fantastic'.

Early days and weeks at home

The return home is an important transition, a marker of progress, but people's reactions can vary at this point. As already described, the neurosurgical unit may have become a 'place of safety' with predictable routines and round-the-clock care, so leaving that behind can sometimes be difficult. Several people described how, in these early days, they were frightened of being left on their own. As Andrew recalled:

> I was actually worried when Wendy [his wife] would disappear out of the room; I didn't want her to go. I didn't want to be left alone. I wanted to know she was nearby. I wanted to know I could get in touch with her, preferably within calling range, and it took a little while for that to ease off. I didn't want to be left in the house on my own. My confidence had gone . . . It was a real blow to me, feeling like that. But eventually it goes.

Although Kaz went to stay with her parents after leaving hospital, she still found she missed the security of being cared for and monitored on the ward:

I felt so secure in hospital because I knew that I was safe in hospital and it was ever so daunting when I came out, even though I was with my parents. I just felt, what if it happens again . . . even if they left the room I'd sit there and think, what if something happened? Because I was ever so slow, and I'd think, what if I needed to go to the toilet quickly and I can't make it?

Tania also went to her parents' home after she left hospital, feeling 'very fragile, very weak', but she also found that she felt:

tentative about everything; scared about doing everything . . . like a cocoon of just wanting to stay safe and not doing very much [but] gradually reintroducing things, maybe coping with more sounds, going for a little walk with my mum and dad, never on my own in the early stages.

Veronica talked about needing someone to 'babysit' her which is quite an appropriate description really. In fact, there were lots of people around and this helped take her mind off the anxieties she was experiencing, but at the same time she was feeling very exhausted. Although these anxieties weren't always very specific, it was not uncommon for people to be frightened that they could have another haemorrhage. As Karen said: 'The thought "Is it going to happen to me again?" started to creep back.' Chapter 9 returns to this theme.

Despite these difficulties, coming home could also be a very positive experience as Lesley found:

The relief of just getting back and knowing I was in my own home was incredible. And I think that was as healing as anything actually. It was about peacefulness [and] I think, to an extent, safety. I just find down here [in a rural area], a very nurturing environment. So I think it was partly that, knowing that I was back in a space where I felt nurtured.

A sense of relief after leaving hospital may be partly related to the 'honeymoon effect' where, in the early stages of recovery, people are just so grateful that they have survived (Buchanan *et al.* 2000). As Lauren described:

After I first came out [of hospital] I was so glad to be alive that I felt very emotional; you suddenly realise how close to death you've been and this creates a wonderful feeling almost of euphoria. I am so glad to be alive, at the same time as having realised that you could go any minute. So you start living in the moment, almost like maybe somebody who is facing death, because you've been that close, so it's a very uplifting and wonderful feeling.

As her recovery progressed, Tania found herself swinging between anxiety and euphoria:

The happiness of recovery was a big, big part . . . Yes, people will feel happy about certain events in their lives but if you haven't got over a traumatic illness or something like this, how do you explain just feeling so joyful just to be alive and just to be happy appreciating small things?

The world of 'not ill, not well'

Twenty years ago, when Faith left hospital, she spent two weeks at the aptly named The Haven – a seaside convalescent home – to continue her recovery. There may be fewer convalescent homes today (though perhaps they have mutated into 'intermediate care facilities'), but they met the need for a halfway house, a stepping stone in recovery. Tania, who went to her parents after leaving hospital, describes her time there as 'like an old-fashioned kind of convalescence'.

This in-between stage of being what might be described as 'not ill but not well' can be frustrating. Despite feeling overwhelmingly tired, Andrew talked of how he 'craved normality. I wanted to be whatever normal is. I wanted it!' Maybe after the crisis of an illness, energy sometimes fades or is depleted:

Crisis generates energy . . . Convalescence is another matter . . . the perceived danger is past, yet the patient isn't able to do much and the little that can be done requires more energy than can be summoned. There are doubts, *Will I ever feel as well as I once did?*

(Osborn 1998: 162, italics in original)

75

Perhaps this is why convalescence can be seen as 'gradual healing (through rest) from illness or injury' – it is gradual and cannot be hurried. Writing about his time in a convalescent home following a major injury, Oliver Sacks describes the uncertainties and the in-between nature of this stage of recovery:

> A peculiar interlude unlike anything we had ever known. We had emerged from . . . the undermining uncertainty about whether we would get well but we had not yet been reclaimed by the daily round of life . . . with its endless obligations, vexations, expectations . . . We were between being 'in' and being 'outside'.
>
> (Sacks 1986: 135)

In these early weeks and months of recovery, energy may be depleted but with enforced inactivity, there is perhaps time – and a space – to start piecing together the events of previous weeks and beginning to understand the impact of having a brain haemorrhage.

Time on your hands

One way of coping with the aftermath of a traumatic event is by distraction, by keeping busy and not allowing oneself to think about it. However, for someone recovering from a brain haemorrhage keeping busy isn't usually an option because physical and mental fatigue means they have to rest. Sleeping will offer some distraction, but many people talked of being unable to read, watch television or follow their previous leisure activities when they got home from hospital. Time is needed for the brain to start healing itself but also for beginning the process of adjusting to post-haemorrhage life:

> Time is a great healer. At both the level of the injured brain and the person's emotional adjustment. It takes time for those damaged neural pathways to gradually re-embroider themselves or to re-connect their broken threads. Similarly it takes time for the new life after head injury to be woven into the material and texture of the old life.
>
> (Powell 2004: 201)

Perhaps this is why Robert McCrum gave his book the title *My Year Off* as it became 'an enforced season of solitude in the midst of a crowded life' (1998: 2). Karen-Ann went to her parents' home to be looked after when she came out of hospital, but recalls how she really wanted to be on her own 'just to think about what had happened because I wasn't having a chance to think about what happened . . . it was – just leave me in peace, just for a little bit'.

Reality dawns

Once people are home again, they have the chance to start piecing together recent events. This is also when it can begin to dawn on them that they have been through a life-threatening experience whose effects will continue to dominate their life for some time to come. This is often when they start to realise how seriously ill they have been. Even if someone was fully conscious and can remember being told they were having a brain haemorrhage, this news can still be difficult to take on board. The communication may be heard but barely digested. The emotional impact may be put on hold. Denial – in this case not allowing oneself to accept the seriousness of the situation – is one strategy for coping with major stressful events of this kind (Carver 1997).

Following a perimesencephalic haemorrhage, John spent three or four days in hospital without asking his family to bring in his pyjamas because, as he wrote: 'I dismissed the idea of needing them – perhaps I thought I wouldn't be in very long.' It was only when he was having an angiogram that he realised, 'the picture on the screen was real and meant I was there on serious business'. When Tania's doctors told her that she'd had a brain haemorrhage, 'because of the fact that I was there alive . . . and talking to people, it didn't connect with the idea of how serious it was . . . it was hard to connect the two together'.

Cracking jokes and making fun of the situation can be an effective coping strategy (Carver 1997), and though she recalls how surreal it felt, her way of coping was to make fun of herself:

With my speech in hospital being so slurry and silly, I used to laugh at it and say to people 'Listen to this!' and read out a few tongue twisters. I don't think other people found it funny but I thought it was hilarious at first.

It was only later that the impact of the haemorrhage seemed less funny:

> With all the attention and all the chaos of being in hospital . . . and being ultra-supported by everyone you think you can cope with whatever happened . . . but it's when you start to think about everyday life and work, you know it's not funny then.

While still in hospital, some people coped by convincing themselves that nothing really serious had happened. When Vernon emerged from a coma, he thinks a nurse told him he'd had a brain haemorrhage but 'I couldn't really think straight . . . couldn't think and remember things for a long time'. Still having no idea why he was in hospital, he also remembers how one of the nurses jokingly told him he was there to have a tooth out. Faced with these two versions of the same event, he decided 'to choose the one that's not so serious'. Karen-Ann knew she was in hospital because she was ill, but thought she'd soon back to normal:

> [But] as soon as I got out of intensive care, that was it. I could be normal. I knew in my mind that I was ill, I knew that there was something wrong with me, but I thought I'd get over it . . . I told my nurse, 'Right, I've had the operation, I can go home now!' and she said 'No, you're not out of the woods yet.'

When someone collapses with a brain haemorrhage and remembers nothing much else for some time, being told you've had a haemorrhage may be almost impossible to take in. Heather recalls being told this: 'I was very shocked and the next thing I did was see my husband and I said to Andy, "Oh my God! They said I've had a brain haemorrhage – there's no way!"'

The mind can protect itself from being overwhelmed by gradually allowing the impact of a traumatic event such as subarachnoid haemorrhage to sink in. Having been told by the neurosurgeon that she'd made an excellent recovery, Lauren agreed and thought she'd 'go home, go back and live a normal life'. But as she recalls: 'I think by the time they released me back to my local hospital, I was beginning to get a sense of the severity of it all.' Although people may begin to take it in, they will often have gaps in the story so part of getting home from hospital may involve piecing together the story so it's a more complete narrative.

Recovering lost time and piecing together the story

People may leave hospital thinking that they have a reasonably clear picture of what has been happening to them, but in a recent study nearly three-quarters of post-haemorrhage patients 'had little clear memory of their first week in hospital' (Pritchard *et al.* 2001: 459). Others may have no memories of several weeks, depending on how gravely ill they have been. Even when people had been given information by their families or by hospital staff, they may either have forgotten this or their version of what happened in hospital is inaccurate (McKenna *et al.* 1989). Filling in these gaps or correcting the distortions at a later date may be helpful (Jarvis 2002).

It may be relatively easy for people to subsequently get hold of factual information. Booklets and other written information can be absorbed at a later date but some people found it difficult to come to terms with 'unremembered time' – the days, or occasionally weeks, which seem to have been completely erased from memory. Specialist nurse Lesley Foulkes sees that for some people '[it's] really hard to get your head around that there was maybe even two days or two months [which] is a blank and you really can't remember it . . . psychologically it just doesn't make sense.'

In the interviews for this book, when people were asked to talk about how the haemorrhage started and what happened while they were in hospital, their accounts were interspersed with 'can't remember', 'don't remember', and 'don't know'. Why does this happen? Shouldn't we have clear memories of such a major event? Lesley Foulkes again:

These bleeds . . . are massively traumatic to the brain and the brain tends at most levels to shut down to doing the essentials; whilst people are aware of what is going on and will often be able to answer in a very sensible fashion, or hold a conversation with you . . . those memories and conversations just aren't stored in the brain because it's just that that's a higher level; the brain is trying to cope with the essentials and the bigger the bleed the worse the patient after the bleed . . . Some of the first levels that appear to go are probably due to the trauma of the bleed in the brain, trying to cope and compensate, to get rid of the non-essentials like storing memories.

People had found various ways of trying to recapture this seemingly lost time. In some cases this was a continuing source of frustration, though others either decided to stop worrying about it or allow other people to piece their story together. Janice remembers very little of the early days in hospital. After coming home, she would think: 'When is this going to come back to me? But then I realise it's pointless to fret over what you can't remember.'

When she arrived at the rehabilitation unit, Jan was unable to remember anything about the previous six weeks. Others have told her what was happening but she's still troubled by her inability to recapture her own memories of that time:

> I can't come to terms with the six weeks from having the haemorrhage to coming round in rehab and it bothers me. People have told me to forget about it, but it's something I can't; I dwell on it, especially when I'm on my own. Everybody's told me everything I've said or done . . . but it's just the not remembering that really bothers me . . . it's like a jigsaw puzzle [and] you're trying to put in the missing pieces! You just want to put those pieces in the jigsaw.

It's as though sometimes other people's memories can't quite compensate for the loss of your own. However, some people pieced the story together by asking family or friends who were around at the time. Although Scott was unable to remember much after he collapsed and was admitted to hospital, as he explained, he is now able to talk about his experiences because 'the story has been told often enough that I do remember'.

When Kaz left hospital to be looked after by her parents, they offered to tell her about her hospital stay: 'There was a lot I didn't know until I came out of hospital and my parents sat me down and said, "This is what happened. If you don't want us to carry on telling you, then just tell us to stop."' This can sometimes be difficult. Learning that several times her parents were urgently summoned to the hospital because she was not expected to live was frightening 'because I thought it was so close . . . and I thought what if it happens again?' However, her father had also written a diary about Kaz's experiences. She was able to read the account over and over again so that their story became her story: 'Fifteen or 16 years on, it's almost like my little story.'

Hearing stories from other people about your time in hospital can be helpful if it contributes to missing parts of the event, but this isn't necessarily so. As specialist nurse Lesley Foulkes explains: 'A lot of people come to [outpatient] clinic and really feel the need to apologise for their behaviour, either from the little snippets they might have patchy memories of, or what they were told they were doing or they were up to . . . this is everyday life for nurses in a neuro unit and there's no need to apologise.' As Lauren discovered, hearing other people's stories about events she's unable to remember herself can be difficult:

Apparently when I came out of the anaesthetic, I tried to pull everything out and get out of the hospital and escape and was quite a handful. My brother-in-law had to come up and calm me down, but I can't remember any of that . . . I find it very disturbing because my sister and brother-in-law tease me about how badly I behaved . . . they can joke about it, but it traumatised me so much, that loss of control or memory.

Despite these gaps in survivors' memories of their time in hospital, there were some events which people remembered quite clearly afterwards, though they were sometimes unsure whether these were dreams or some kind of hallucination (probably caused by the haemorrhage and/or medication). These generally didn't seem to bother people. Sometimes they could find explanations for them, sometimes they didn't, but they are included here as it may reassure others that these are actually 'normal' experiences:

I had some very very peculiar dreams . . . one was being on a trolley in the very first hospital I'd worked at . . . somebody was pushing me like hell over the cobbles . . . very bizarre . . . [and] meeting my Uncle Ken who I'd never met before because he was dead before I was ever born! Then coming round a bit and thinking my consultant was my Uncle Ken! . . . and of course, there was lots of tubing . . . and I can remember clearly saying 'What are you putting the vacuum cleaner on me for?'

(Pam)

81

I used to wake up and I'd see if someone's bed was there opposite me and I'd be on top of that one over there – upright! I'm standing upright watching him down there. This is the hallucination I was having . . . I was having quite a few. It's all these tablets, I think.

(James)

The next thing I remember [after the coiling] I was there myself . . . the neurological people wear a royal blue [uniform] with a yellow stripe down each side and I had one on. And this face-less person alongside me had one on as well and there was a series of doors and this faceless person just said to me 'You go through that one.' And I went through it.

(Roy)

6

LOOKING FOR HELP

Depending on the initial outcome of their haemorrhage, people will
have differing needs for information, advice, support and rehabilitation services. This chapter describes the kinds of help they had
but also what they would like to have received after leaving hospital. Recent research has drawn attention to the importance of
effective follow-up (e.g. Buchanan *et al.* 2000; Pritchard *et al.* 2001,
2004; Kirkness *et al.* 2002; Powell *et al.* 2002, 2004; Jarvis and
Talbot 2004), but the reality is that this is by no means routinely
available to people leaving hospital. There is still too often 'a hiatus
in care and support by community-based services' (Pritchard *et al.*
2001: 456), although sometimes people were able to find help
themselves – through web-based message boards, for example.

This chapter describes people's experience of looking for information and advice, mutual support through contact with other
survivors, their use of the internet for information, advice and
support, the role of support groups, the provision of specialist
nurses, GPs' involvement and community-based and outpatient
services.

Information and advice

Apart from survivors sometimes needing services such as speech
therapy and physiotherapy, people frequently mentioned that they
wanted information about subarachnoid haemorrhage and what to
expect during their recovery. They wanted to know if what they
were experiencing was 'normal', whether their recovery was pro-
ceeding within expected timescales, and whether they could expect
to make a complete recovery. They had many many questions.

When specialist nurse Anne Jarvis interviewed a small group of
patients about their experiences of recovery, her findings confirmed

that people are left wanting to discover and understand more about what has been happening to them. They not only wanted general factual information but also had questions relating specifically to their situation:

> It seems [they] have a thirst for knowledge and information, and it might be useful for the specialist nurse to provide factual information and current known statistical information about the risk of recurrence plus answers to any other questions posed by the patient and family.
>
> (Jarvis 2002: 1436)

When Wendy was leaving hospital she received very little advice and information about recovery:

> because they just said everybody's different. It was a case really of just 'Go home, see how you get on and do what you can do', which wasn't very helpful . . . when you're a couple of weeks down the line and you start thinking I'm not making very much progress. What should I be doing? Is this normal? It's at this point you need information.

Some neurosurgery units give patients and their families a booklet about subarachnoid haemorrhage and recovery (e.g. Brain and Spine Foundation 2002, 2005b; Foulkes 2004). Wessex Neurological Centre has produced a DVD of patients' experiences of subarachnoid haemorrhage (2007). People were sometimes also given information about the Brain and Spine Foundation's telephone helpline.

Megan appreciated being given some written information by the hospital: 'I thought the booklet was excellent and I did refer to [it] a lot. I kept sort of flicking [through] it.' Despite this, there were other things she wanted to know. She would like to have had a picture of the clip inserted during surgery and to find out whether it could become loose. (This is highly unlikely to happen, but it doesn't stop people worrying about it so there's a need for both information and reassurance.)

Janet found some patient and carer leaflets were helpful – but she only got hold of them by chance when, two months after she left hospital, they were handed to her by a visiting researcher. As she wrote: 'It would have been nice to have been given them on discharge.' Patients were generally given verbal information during their hospital stay, but as Lesley said: 'If you're told too much, it's not going to be very useful.' Even if, as is often the case, relatives are also given verbal information, being in the midst of a traumatic event they too may be unable to take it in and remember what they've been told.

Neurological conditions (such as subarachnoid haemorrhage) are diagnosed and treated following an acute episode, when patients are unable to assimilate much information, so information and support will be needed in the following weeks and months (Collett *et al.* 2006). This is echoed by others who suggest that information about the haemorrhage and about the emotional consequences should be repeated a few weeks after the event (Sheldrick *et al.* 2006). There may also be simply too much to assimilate on one occasion. Christine's experiences bear this out. While still in hospital, she remembers being given a lot of information but was unable to retain it: 'Often people would say things and I realise now that I wasn't taking anything in . . . the only thing they were concerned about was physical things.' She was also given a lot of instructions by one of the doctors, but it was only about four weeks after leaving hospital that she was able to remember them.

Although general information and advice is available from a number of different sources, people often had questions about their individual situation (Pritchard *et al.* 2001). As Karen found:

> The [Salford and Wessex web] site was very good but it wasn't sometimes giving me enough information . . . I wanted to know a bit more as I was getting better. The booklet was good but it was very basic; it was the sort of stuff you left hospital with because probably that's all that your brain could cope with.

There was also a recurring theme of people wanting information and advice from another person, rather than having to rely solely on written materials. Face-to-face contact – or at least a voice on the end of the telephone – really seemed to matter. In the light of the considerable levels of anxiety experienced by so many people (see pp. 130–35), there was perhaps a need for direct reassurance – to feel that 'everything would be okay'.

Because Patsy moved from a specialist unit to a different hospital, she seems to have slipped through the net, leaving her without the kind of support she would like to have had:

> I think support would have been nice; just someone saying to me, 'Well, this is normal and you can't expect to be any different.' I think we all don't know . . . whether this is how it's going to be forever? But there was nobody; I had nobody to turn to at all, not anywhere . . . What support can they give you? It's just someone to talk to, isn't it really?

People seem to need information and advice, but a significant proportion also need psychological support, particularly after they leave hospital. As Christine said: 'There was no looking at my state of mind or anything like that.' And Karen 'didn't find that there was anybody looking after my mental welfare'. The Brain and Spine Foundation, whose telephone helpline is staffed by neuro-science health professionals, has found that nearly three-quarters of their callers are patients and although most were looking for information (e.g. the foundation's publications), over a quarter were phoning for emotional support (Collett *et al.* 2006).

Meeting other survivors

When people were asked what information, advice and support they wanted after leaving hospital, they frequently mentioned wanting to meet other people who'd survived a subarachnoid haemorrhage. Even when people had returned home to supportive family and friends, there was still this wish – this need even? – to have some kind of contact with people who had been through a similar experience. While still in hospital they may have already been part of what Oliver Sacks (1986) describes as the 'fellowship' of patients. After leaving that behind, people were often looking for reassurance, for hope of recovery, and less of a sense of isolation.

Veronica had kept in touch with one or two people she'd met in hospital – 'comparing notes and seeing how other people feel' – and others may do this, or may be able to join a support group, but many others were more isolated. On the hospital ward everyone is, to some extent, in the same boat, but at home, Patsy recalled, she was 'feeling very isolated when I came out . . . I'm sent home . . . and nothing, nothing at all'. This sense of isolation is echoed by another survivor's experience: 'Doctors blithely say you'll be off work three or four months without thinking of the consequences – it was like being banished to a desert island, only there was nothing nice about it; it was an island of desolation' (Pritchard *et al.* 2001: 461).

Even after his physical recovery was well under way, Vernon still felt he was something of an outsider – somehow different from other people: 'I felt alienated still and didn't feel that I was like everybody else.' Joining a local Headway group helped to lessen that sense of alienation: 'The only people that I felt I was like were the people at Headway, the groups at Headway.' After being a 'client', he then became a volunteer and subsequently worked for them for a time as an assistant manager.

Fellow survivors not only have experiences in common, but they can also offer hope. Six months after his stroke, Robert McCrum met Donal O'Kelly, a founder of Different Strokes, which in turn led to meetings with other younger stroke survivors:

> [It was] comforting to be in the company of those who'd experienced and understood what I'd just been through . . . I was terribly lost and lonely and was glad to hear from someone who seemed not only to understand how I was feeling, but who also offered a ray of hope for the future.
>
> (McCrum 1998: 197–8)

Meeting other survivors who can offer hope can be particularly important in the early stages of their recovery. Through informal networking, Megan was able to talk to people soon after coming out of hospital and she'd like to see these kinds of opportunities made more widely available:

> Often at that stage, you just want to see somebody who had it last year and is doing well, because it gives you a boost, doesn't it, to speak to somebody that actually has had it happen to them. And sometimes it's nicer to talk to a person than latch on to a computer . . . When I had mine done, somebody gave me Veronica's phone number and I rang her and it was great! And then somebody said, 'Oh, we know somebody who had that done. He's happy to talk to you. Ring him up!' So I rang him . . . And it's great, this sort of networking of people, during the acute phase when you think, oh good, people *do* get better from it. And this is why I think that it's something else that people can turn to, to make them realise that, yes, you can get on with your life. And I was very

conscious of the fact that when I came out of hospital I wanted
to talk to people that have had it and recovered.

Although Rosie already belongs to a support group, she has also
been in touch with another survivor who lives some distance from
her in a rural area with little in the way of support. She'd like to see
more opportunities for this kind of mutual support:

> Having somebody you can talk to, somebody that's been there
> and done that and somebody that understands. If you say, 'It's
> like walking around on foam rubber' and the other person says
> 'Oh, I had that!' you suddenly feel so much better because you
> don't feel that this is something serious, or something isolated;
> it's something that somebody else understands. So I think that
> some sort of database . . . where people can phone you, contact
> you or contact your group for help, is such a good idea.

Neurological centres often admit patients from a wide catchment
area, so that attending a support group can be impracticable. In
Wessex, in addition to their support group meetings, specialist
nurse Lesley Foulkes and her colleagues have set up a contact
network to link up patients with each other. Ex-patients who agree
to participate will supply the information they are happy to have
given out and can then access the database to find other people.
They may be looking for someone of a similar age, someone living
near them, or someone with a similar problem. Contact can be by
phone, by email or they can arrange to meet up.

Unless they are in touch with others in a similar situation, people
may want to know whether they are recovering fast enough –
perhaps they are seeking a kind of affirmation? Although everyone's pace of recovery will be different, this doesn't stop people
wanting to know, wanting some kind of confirmation that they are
doing all right. As Karen-Ann found, being told by her GP, her
neurosurgeon and her friends that she was making good progress
wasn't enough to reassure her because, she said, 'I had nothing to
benchmark myself against!' Coming out of hospital, when she was
very weak and finding it difficult to walk, Kaz was also looking for
benchmarks:

At that point, I didn't know how long it was going to be that I was going to stay like that; it would have been nice to have been able to speak to someone and they could have said to me 'Well the same thing happened to me and it took so long' or someone could say 'Well, I'm still like that now after' . . . I didn't know what to expect the recovery process would be.

A survivor of brain haemorrhage may feel that they're the only person this has ever happened to, but discovering that this isn't the case can be reassuring. As Andrew said: 'I think we all crave to talk to people who've had a similar experience and then I found it, strangely, at work: some people came out of the woodwork to say "Well, actually I had that twenty years ago".' A month or two after his haemorrhage, John too came across a fellow survivor – another doctor who'd been treated by coiling and had successfully returned to work – which 'made me feel a little less alone with it'.

No two people's experiences will be exactly the same, but if it doesn't sound too contradictory, there will be points of shared experiences and common concerns. Andrew has been offering support to another survivor:

It's been good to talk . . . I'm sure they feel they're talking to someone who's experienced it at least – it's maybe not the same, but it's someone who knows what it's all about.

Using the internet

The internet has multiple potential uses. It can provide people with ways of meeting others recovering from subarachnoid haemorrhage, enable them to access information about haemorrhages and strokes and obtain advice about recovery and sources of further help such as support groups. The internet plays an increasingly important part in people's lives today. Over 50 per cent of UK adults now have broadband at home, a sevenfold increase over the last four years (OFCOM 2007). This has significant implications for survivors. Many will be spending protracted periods of time at home, so it is hardly surprising if they and their families turn to the internet, particularly, though not exclusively, if they have mobility or communication difficulties or are geographically isolated. The World Wide Web also enables people in the UK and further afield to have contact with each other by participating in a virtual support group (Down *et al.* 2005).

People usually link up with each other by using message boards or discussion forums. Although internet users aren't limited to UK-based sites, in practice people were using the Brain and Spine Foundation's online discussion forum and/or Wessex and Great Manchester Neuroscience Centres' message board (though the latter ceased to operate in 2006). A new online support group (www.behindthegray.net) was also set up in 2006, as 'an online community for those whose lives or relatives/friends have been affected by subarachnoid haemorrhage or stroke'. Some people have also used online support from organisations such as Different Strokes (for younger stroke survivors) and the Stroke Association's TalkStroke discussion forum (see Appendix B).

The majority of these message boards are moderated. Messages are first emailed to a moderator for their approval before being posted on the internet for others to read. Peer support groups are sometimes unmoderated or there may be insufficient resources to scrutinise every single message, but a recent review of online peer-to-peer support groups found no evidence that virtual communities can harm people (Eysenbach *et al.* 2004). Message boards or discussion forums enable people to share their experiences, to get and give support and to share coping strategies. For Janet, finding a support group discussion page on the internet was very reassuring because 'it helped a great deal to find out other sufferers had the same fears and concerns as myself'. Karen also found participating in a message board was 'an absolute godsend'. As she says: 'I really feel you need to be able to talk to fellow sufferers and share experiences. When I've had down days, there's always been somebody to share it with and vice versa, there's always somebody worse off than you.' Since then, she has been instrumental in setting up an online support group (www.behindthegray.net).

Online peer support can be personally empowering, enabling people to use their knowledge and experience in a positive manner, although it is worth pointing out that advice based on one person's experience may not always be appropriate for someone else. This potential drawback is, however, outweighed by the benefits it can offer to those who may have no other sources of help and guidance. Vernon used the internet, including Different Strokes and the Brain and Spine Foundation sites, to research activities and strategies which could help with his physical and psychological recovery:

I tried everything really . . . anything and everything, . . . talking to other people about what they've done . . . just having that open mind and thinking, okay, maybe that will be good, maybe that won't be. [And] I would get lots of messages back, saying 'Well, I've got this problem; has anyone got an suggestions or anything'.

Apart from accessing peer support and advice, the other main reason why people used the internet was to find out about subarachnoid haemorrhage and recovery. Organisations such as the Brain and Spine Foundation and Salford NHS Trust's subarachnoid haemorrhage site offer accurate and patient-friendly information, but a general search for 'subarachnoid haemorrhage' will produce additional information, sometimes aimed at professional rather than lay audiences. For Christine:

It's like the internet to me has been the world library in your house . . . that's been a lot of help, just finding out . . . reading research papers as well [and] even though you can usually only get the abstract [i.e. summary], it gives you conclusions and things like that.

Although Christine has found it helpful, perhaps using the internet to get hold of information should come with a health warning? People's experiences were sometimes rather mixed. As Scott found: 'Although it's a great tool, it can be very scary when you're having a critical illness because [of] the morbidity rates and all the rest of it. I think they're very scary things to look at.' Like Scott, Veronica admits that she was nervous about what she might read on the internet: 'I was frightened that I would hear something sort of negative or something that was going to make me worry.'

Lauren came home from hospital and went straight onto the internet but, she recalls: 'I started to realise how bad it was and how much at risk I still was . . . until the blood cleared out of my brain.' Lauren was already aware that her father had died of a brain haemorrhage and she decided to stop her internet searches at that point, feeling too frightened about what she had already read. Karen also came home from hospital with many questions but no one she could turn to at that point who could provide some answers so she turned to the internet:

> At this point I started madly researching on the internet – SAH, coiling, seizures. It seemed to be the only way for me to access the information I was looking for. I read every article that I could, often regretting the outcome of what I read. Maybe ignorance is bliss but sometimes I also felt that knowledge was power.

As Karen said, 'knowledge is power', but is that knowledge necessarily accurate? When David started looking for information and advice, he was aware that 'you can pick up a lot of bad information on the internet as well as good information'.

So, like it or not, people used – and will continue to use – the internet. Maybe they should take the following advice from the *British Medical Journal* that 'before we conclude that the information on the net is inadequate, incomplete and generally scary, we might try comparing it with what the typical doctor tells the typical patient in the typical 10-minute [appointment]' (*BMJ* Editorial 2002: 555).

Support groups

A recent review of subarachnoid haemorrhage suggests that survivors 'need information about support groups' (Al-Shahi *et al.* 2006). That's certainly the case: support groups provide opportunities for people to meet others who are on the same journey of recovery, although there are currently very few groups specifically for subarachnoid haemorrhage survivors (see Appendix C). Several people had joined groups run by Headway (for people with head injuries) or Different Strokes (for younger stroke victims). Specialist nurse Lesley Foulkes describes the support group she runs, which was set up because patients and their families wanted to meet others in a similar situation:

> The main focus is for people to be able to have an opportunity to meet with somebody else who's been through a similar experience and to be able to share experiences, anxieties, ideas, whatever. Family members can share experiences of living with somebody who's had a haemorrhage.
>
> It's also a resource and an information point. We try and run it that half the meetings are more formal and

information-led, so we talk about specifics; people who've had a haemorrhage don't really remember that operation they've had and what went on, and then [there are] familial concerns or things like that.

Then the other half of the meetings is very much informal where it's up to the group what they want to do and it's much more just greet and talk to each other . . . People know that they can come if they want to, but it's not like an appointment they've go to turn up to.

They know we [the two specialist nurses] will be there and if there are questions and concerns they can just take you to one side [and ask you].

So it's three things: actual formal information; having someone there to maybe answer questions; but the main focus is to share experiences.

For Andrew, attending a support group was:

an invaluable thing – to go and realise that you weren't on your own, that other people experienced similar things, that there was hope . . . and that there was support. Just talking to someone else who's experienced it makes a huge difference.

Although the group Jan attends includes people with more severe disabilities, she discovered she still could learn from other members. She also finds the group reassuring and supportive because 'it gives me a bit more calmness'. David and his wife joined a support group three months after his haemorrhage and he finds it helps his recovery in many different ways:

Absolutely fantastic . . . you meet new friends, and you can exchange your own things that have happened, your own experiences . . . and [the specialist nurse] is there if you have any problems. . . . And it's a place to let your frustrations out, to let your true feelings and emotions out, because, I think . . . sometimes your family (I'm not saying they do) can get a bit bored.

People are sometimes anxious about whether they are doing well enough or how they compare with other survivors, but in practice having a group that includes people at different stages of recovery can be helpful. Lesley Foulkes again:

> We have people who come who've had a haemorrhage eight weeks ago and there's somebody who had a haemorrhage four years ago, so they don't make direct comparisons, and the people from four years ago, I think they find it therapeutic being able to offer their experience to the newer people and the newer people find it very reassuring to see somebody who's that bit further down the line; to see where they're at now and to see how they got there, so we don't seem to have too much of 'Oh you're doing so much better than me' because people are at varying stages.

Holding support group meetings at the neurosurgical unit can be difficult for some people when the unit holds difficult or traumatic memories. As Lesley Foulkes has found, some people are unable to attend the support group as it has too many negative and difficult associations. Fortunately this isn't always the case. When he first came out of hospital, Scott enjoyed returning for support group meetings (and outpatient appointments): 'The trips . . . were a big deal for me. I don't know why but it was the place where I'd been for so long . . . I did feel happier down here than at home.'

Specialist nurses

As well as working with patients on the wards, specialist nurses also have a key part to play as the bridge between hospital and home. Although some people are fortunate enough to be supported by one of these nurses, they are still a scarce resource in the UK, with only a handful of neurocentres having one or more specialist subarachnoid haemorrhage nurses. The benefits of employing specialist nurses – including the financial savings – are clear. In one region, it was found that when people had early and easy access to a specialist liaison nurse they had reduced time off work, fewer readmissions and needed less time with medical staff (Pritchard *et al.* 2004: 17). For someone like Rosie, who had ongoing contact with a specialist nurse, she 'couldn't have done without her . . . she rang me up very soon after I got home and to know that there was someone there to ask questions was really helpful'. Being able to contact someone who has specialist knowledge is invaluable, particularly in the early stages of recovery when what are often relatively minor worries or concerns can be addressed before they escalate into becoming major concerns.

Like Rosie, David found the contact with a specialist nurse has been very helpful. Perhaps because he became ill and was treated outside the UK, he only found this support after some delay:

> It was like a black cloud had just been lifted off us. All the questions we asked were answered 110 per cent and it was absolutely brilliant, but I could have done with it two months earlier. [If] we have any problems, I can ring her up . . . especially when I kept on getting these headaches and I kept on being sick . . . and she'd say 'Don't worry; it's all part and parcel; just take it easy.'

Of course headaches and vomiting are frightening and worrying – they replicate the symptoms which commonly occur at the time of the haemorrhage – but it's not always easy to know what is 'normal'. If people are treated in one area but move to a completely different area to recover, like David, it may be some time before they find out about the specialist nurses. Tania, like David, only learned that specialist nurse support and a support group were available two months after she left hospital:

> It was fantastic. It was a real relief to see the agenda [in the support group] of things they talked about and to have her available on the phone as well . . . it was really helpful to have face-to-face contact.

For Rosie, David and others who are in the same area, the specialist nurses run a support group but also offer telephone support.

Although the specialist nurse's role may vary slightly from area to area, the help they may offer can address many of the needs of patients and their families and can include:

- supporting the patient and their family during the hospital stay, providing information and explanations, and answering their questions
- providing written information about subarachnoid haemorrhage and recovery, and contact details (email and telephone number) for the specialist nurse service

- phoning people within the first few weeks after their discharge to see how things are going
- having subsequent contact, depending on the patient's progress and their needs in recovery
- seeing the patient in the outpatient clinic which is led by specialist nurses unless further surgery is required
- supporting the GP and healthcare professionals who are non-specialists in neurology/neurosurgery, by acting as a specialist resource
- identifying patients with psychological problems which may require referral to neuropsychology services.

(Jarvis and Talbot 2004; Pritchard *et al.* 2004)

The role of the GP

Some people were advised by the hospital to contact their GP after they returned home, although others who didn't get this advice were uncertain about whether they should see their GP and what the GP's role could or should be during their recovery. Experiences varied, with some having little to do with their GP, while others' GPs were more involved with their post-hospital care. The main issues raised during the interviews were: the GP's role as a non-specialist in relation to subarachnoid haemorrhage; how GPs cared for their post-haemorrhage patients, and communication between the GP and specialist health services.

How often can a GP expect to see patients who've had a subarachnoid haemorrhage? A full-time GP with a caseload of 2000 patients can expect to see one such patient about every seven or eight years (van Gjin *et al.* 2007). Others have suggested that a GP may see six to eight such patients during their entire career (Pritchard *et al.* 2001). So these patients do not form a regular part of a GP's caseload. Given this situation, GPs have few opportunities to develop any substantial knowledge or experience of working with patients recovering from subarachnoid haemorrhage. As David said: 'He's an absolutely fantastic doctor, but he's only a GP and this is a specialist thing.' Brian pointed out: 'If you have a cold and you want to know what colour Tunes to have, then go to a doctor, he can help you. Anything more serious, you need to find someone else.' And Patsy, whose GP only came to see her when her husband asked for a home visit, said: 'I feel a GP is more used to seeing coughs and colds and such, and suddenly there I am, I've had all this stuff. He probably looked at me and thought, well, I don't quite know what to do with her really.' Little wonder that only 40 per cent of the people interviewed by Pritchard and his colleagues (2001) felt that their GP knew enough about sub-arachnoid haemorrhage to provide care.

Even though GPs may have little knowledge or experience of subarachnoid haemorrhage, their patients appreciated it when their GP made it their business to go away and learn more about it. In Rosie's case: '[My GP] didn't know very much, but she was obviously interested, and the second time I saw her, she'd obviously been reading up about it.' Scott also had a GP who admitted he wasn't a specialist but was prepared to learn more: 'I can't sing his praises highly enough . . . he came round the first time and said he didn't know a lot about subarachnoid haemorrhage but he'd certainly go and find out – and he did.'

Although maybe people would have preferred their GP to have at least some knowledge or expertise, sometimes the roles were reversed and it was the GP who was learning from them. As Wendy found: 'He'd never come across anybody with a subarach-noid haemorrhage, so he was a nice chap but he was pretty much learning from me – which is good for him but not so good for me!' Christine's GP was in his forties and had never previously met a patient with subarachnoid haemorrhage but, as she says: 'The surgery, you can't fault it. They've been fantastic [but] you can't expect a doctor to know in-depth. I always felt I knew more than him in the end!'

As part of the primary care service, GPs are the gatekeepers to specialist or secondary care, so there were times when people needed their GP to liaise with neurological or other specialist services. In John's case that worked well: 'My GP was very helpful in being supportive, always directive when he needed to be, and facilitative in referring me to the physician for anti-hypertension treatment review.' In Brian's case, the primary–secondary care interface worked less well. After being signed off by the hospital for three months, when it came to renewing his sickness certification his GP practice and the hospital where he was treated were appar-ently unable to agree whose responsibility this was.

If the haemorrhage started with a sudden collapse people usually (though not always) went directly to hospital by ambulance, but others will have been to see their GP – sometimes repeatedly over weeks or longer – but without being referred for further investi-gations before the haemorrhage occurred. It was hardly surprising therefore that people could have mixed feelings about going back to see their GP after they left hospital. However, it was possible to put this behind them. As Lesley said: 'Water under the bridge! I'm not left feeling angry or bitter about it; it's just really a comment that I think they missed something there; and I also missed something by not going to my optician.' As Janice, who'd had a previous haemorrhage 22 years ago, explained:

> I was less than pleased with my GP, after him ignoring when I went to see him with double vision and headaches! He said, 'We'll see how you are in a week or so' during which time the aneurysm ruptured and he left me in mortal danger. But I haven't given him a hard time about it. I've never made a fuss about it; I think, what's the point, it's not going to change what happened.

People sometimes described their GP as 'supportive' which perhaps meant that they were offering reassurance when needed – and reassurance from a health professional could be just what was needed. Kaz's experience illustrates this well:

> I was getting headaches and of course I got worried so my mum took me down to the GP and they just assured me that they'd looked at the notes and there was nothing to worry about it and that I would get headaches after [the haemorrhage] . . . she was very good. She said, 'If you've ever got any worries, just come down; don't worry about an appointment, just come down and see me.'

The importance of offering reassurance after someone leaves hospital shouldn't be underestimated. Anxiety is common – particularly when people are scared that the onset of a headache means they're having another haemorrhage (see pp. 113–14, 130–1) – but it may not always be easy for GPs to decide when to refer someone back to hospital and when to offer reassurance (McKenna et al. 1989). For Vernon, his GP provided good medical care but also made time to listen to him respectfully:

> He's a brilliant doctor, a fantastic doctor. I was really lucky to have such a good doctor. He would give me lots of time and

look everything up . . . he would sit down and talk to me about it and then try and work out maybe, what the best sort of tablets might be, which tablets are agreeing or disagreeing with me, looking up stuff on his screen . . . and sit down and have a good chat about everything . . . [and] just sort of value me as a person.

Roy is someone who, even though he didn't need a great deal of medical after-care, had a GP who kept an eye on his recovery:

I said to her 'I've had a subarachnoid haemorrhage and I've been told not many of you doctors have seen one of these before.' And she said to me, 'I've seen loads of them when I was a locum so I can help you as much as you like!' And she was very supportive, very good. I popped in to see her about every couple of weeks or so and she just took my blood pressure and we had a chat and that was it basically. . . . She just kept an eye on me really.

Perhaps Roy's and Vernon's experiences point to the kind of follow-up which everyone should be able to access during their recovery?

Community-based and outpatient services

Survivors need access to multidisciplinary teams who can screen for and manage any physical, cognitive and emotional difficulties likely to affect their recovery (Jarvis and Talbot 2004; Al-Shahi *et al.* 2006). These kinds of services are likely to include neuropsychology, physiotherapy, speech therapy and occupational therapy. Specialist nurses and support groups also have an important part to play. Follow-up services need to be tailored to each person's individual circumstances so that they can be helped to re-engage with daily living activities and regain their independence (Powell *et al.* 2004). In practice, patients' follow-up was often rather haphazard (Jarvis and Talbot 2004), sometimes no more than an outpatient clinic appointment at a future date. It didn't appear to be routine practice for people to be assessed and offered a structured package of care when they left hospital (unless they were transferred to a residential rehabilitation centre).

99

It is not uncommon for people to be discharged from hospital without the prearranged support services they need. Pam returned home following a haemorrhagic stroke which had left her with significant physical and cognitive difficulties, but she and her husband had to be proactive in order for her to get the services she needed:

> There was nothing on discharge. I was discharged and that was that. I was still ill; I couldn't walk properly. I couldn't distinguish between a television and a computer and the microwave. My memory was absolutely atrocious and my speech on occasions practically non-existent . . . I could have done with going somewhere else prior to being discharged from hospital, just to get myself back together again. At that time my mobility was very poor. I was staggering and falling. I don't know how we actually got physio[therapy] in the end but we managed to get it. My speech was appalling. We managed to get speech therapy and I still can't remember how.

Scott, on the other hand, was able to get help from the neuro-rehabilitation team in his area:

> I had every support that you could possibly imagine! They have a neuro team in [his local area] and although they were very busy, they get round to you eventually. We had a team. We had the neuro-physio[therapist] and my occupational therapist [who] referred me to the clinical neuropsychologist. I had the full works!

Although Scott had to wait a month or two before receiving these services, Tania left hospital with a planned package of support services, having already been assessed during her inpatient stay:

> I had already been referred to a speech therapist and an occupational therapist and a physiotherapist and I'd been seen by hospital-based therapists for those three things, in the hospital, I had sessions with them all and checks. And they'd all referred me on . . . so I knew there was a programme and a plan . . . which was reassuring.

Several people had used neuropsychology services, for help with cognitive problems or emotional difficulties – or sometimes both. Tania's speech therapist referred her to a neuropsychologist:

> She's helped every step really . . . it's been an emotional support and then the reassurance of having the testing . . . all the therapies have been key in my recovery but that one has been the most consistently helpful for me. She identified to start with that anxiety was probably the key thing that she could help me to address and we started off with relaxation techniques . . . I've done things before like that in my working life . . . but I think when you're in this really serious position where you are really traumatised [that] you really see the value of these techniques. After she'd dealt with the anxiety, that was ongoing anyway . . . we moved on to looking at thought challenging . . . [to] help me approach some worries differently.

Others had also used cognitive psychologists who were able to work with them on challenging and reframing their thoughts and beliefs which can often be very negative after a haemorrhage. Graham, for example, found it gave him 'a different way of looking at things'. Andrew also had some cognitive counselling which helped him manage his return to work, but he has since moved to another counsellor to address some emotional issues.

In addition to clinical psychology services, counsellors and psychotherapists can also support people in addressing the emotional difficulties which they may be experiencing in recovery (e.g. Buchanan *et al.* 2000; Morris *et al.* 2004; Larner 2005). Pam was already seeing a therapist and had started counselling training when she had her haemorrhage. Six weeks after returning home, she returned to her therapist where she could start to take on board what had happened and then begin to make plans for the future:

> [It] was a case of, I've just had a brain haemorrhage – what is going on? I'm not crying! Where are my emotions? I'm frightened; I know I'm frightened and what I've done is to try and reassure other people that things are okay – and they're not really okay . . . I think initially it was just to have that supporting 'other', just to be there and say, well, Pam, it *has* happened to you. And not having somebody there who was telling me it was

going to be all right and 'Yes, you look wonderful' . . . It was okay not to be okay. And then it got on to, well, you say you want to do A, B, C, D – how are you going to achieve it?

Wendy went to counselling to help her cope with depression but she also sees a homeopath and a herbalist, which she chose in preference to using antidepressant medication.

7

PHYSICAL AND SENSORY EFFECTS

Introduction

This book focuses on psychosocial recovery, but although detailed information about physical and sensory problems was not gathered during the interviews, people described how these had affected their recovery. Carleen Scott's study of quality of life following subarachnoid haemorrhage found the impact was considerable:

> Issues such as constant headaches or migraines, unstable balance, poor vision, not being able to walk as far as before the SAH, not being able to exercise, excessive tiredness, losing the strength from the side of the body. These appear to be very common effects of an SAH. All these issues were ranked in the top four ways the SAH had affected participants' lives.
>
> (C.R. Scott 2006: 34)

The extent of physical and sensory difficulties will vary from person to person, although recovery can sometimes continue over quite lengthy periods of time:

> Many people recover completely, but in some cases, the damage to brain tissue may, for example, cause speech disturbance, weakness down one side, or double vision. However, not all damage is permanent and these problems can continue to improve over a number of years.
>
> (Brain and Spine Foundation 2002: 15)

Sometimes problems will not disappear completely, but as this and other chapters illustrate, people had often found ways of adapting to them and continuing to lead satisfying lives.

The remainder of this chapter focuses on the following: physical mobility; eyesight; epilepsy; fatigue; sleep disturbance; headaches and head pain; sense of taste and smell; unexplained physical sensations; changed physical appearance.

Mobility

A subarachnoid haemorrhage can affect physical mobility in varying degrees, ranging from a slight weakness in the legs and arms to a complete loss of power. Although it's impossible to predict whether recovery will be complete, with the physiotherapy and an exercise plan the limbs will often gradually recover strength (Foulkes 2004; Brain and Spine Foundation 2005b). Mobility problems can range from needing to use (often temporarily) a wheelchair, to general unsteadiness.

Both Karen and Vernon were initially wheelchair users. While he was still in hospital, a doctor told Vernon: 'Unfortunately you'll be wheelchair bound for the rest of your life.' He wasn't going to accept this prognosis because 'that sort of made me think, No! I'm not going to do that; I'm not going to spend the rest of my life [in a wheelchair] I'm only 28!' Although having also been told that most of his physical recovery would occur within the first couple of months, he decided otherwise: 'Four months after the brain haemorrhage I knew that I could still rehabilitate more.' Learning how to walk again was a priority when he got home. A combination of dizzy spells and problems with her eyesight significantly affected Karen's mobility:

> It never stopped me from going out. I didn't really care what people thought. I mean, I was in a wheelchair. I used to think, oh, you shouldn't really be in here – I feel a bit of a fraud . . . there's so many people worse off than me . . . but looking back now, that was crazy to even think about it. I couldn't walk and that was it.

Although she no longer needs her wheelchair, physical problems continue to affect her: 'I think it's been a combination of having the dizzy spells and the eyesight, so my balance is out and I just can't walk very far and I've found that really frustrating and quite upsetting really.'

Even if people no longer need to use a wheelchair, they may still not want to rely on a walking stick outside the home. After a spell of inpatient rehabilitation, Patsy was determined not to come home with a Zimmer frame, but she still felt self-conscious about going out with her stick: 'I can remember going to town for the first time with it and I just thought – No! I'm not walking with it – it draws attention to you!' When her husband pointed out that she was still unable to walk properly and people were bumping into her, she agreed because 'from that point of view it was good, but I just felt everyone was looking at me so I didn't use [the stick] for long!'

Other people, however, may find that carrying a walking stick provides some protection. When Rosie no longer really needed her stick for going out she missed it because 'it was a symbol to everybody around me that there was something not quite right'. Though there is often considerable improvement over time, full recovery may not always be possible. Roy finds there are ups and downs when it comes to walking: 'Some days I can walk reasonably well and other days, hopeless . . . like cramp without the pain. The muscles just don't want to work . . . and that's affected the quality of life for me.'

Lesley, on the other hand, has been able to return to her previous enjoyment of walking and mushroom gathering. For the first two months she was unable to go for walks: 'It took quite a bit of time to get back into that . . . actually it took a year probably before physically I felt reasonably okay and was walking at my normal pace again, rather than plodding along.' Apart from physical problems, fatigue can also affect how well someone walks. Three years after her haemorrhage, Wendy still finds this is the case:

When I get very tired, I act as if I'm drunk. I still have problems walking. I can't walk in a straight line and I will mix words up . . . that's how my family know I'm getting tired because they say 'You get this glazed look on your face and you start walking off that way', or I become a bit manic and I scuttle along. I don't know I'm doing it, but apparently that's what I do!

Eyesight

After subarachnoid haemorrhage, vision can be affected in several different ways, ranging from sore eyes to permanent double vision or blurring. These difficulties will obviously have a direct effect on people's quality of life. They can determine when and whether they return to driving, they can affect general mobility, indoors and out, and make activities like reading very difficult. Twenty years after her haemorrhage, Faith still suffers from double vision, apart from a brief period following surgery to restore normal vision, after which the double vision returned. Although she still manages to get out and about, since the haemorrhage she's never been able to return to books though reading had been something she really enjoyed. As she explains: 'It's not simply a question of reading the words, it's actually having enough energy left to take in the meaning. You can't do the two at once!'

Kaz was also left with problems with her eyesight, including double vision. She isn't worried that this put an end to the driving lessons she was having at the time, but it did affect her day-to-day life, although she's learned to adapt to double vision:

> So every now and then, if I get tired, then my right eye might start to wander a little bit. So I'm looking at the clock now, I know what is the clock and what is double vision, whereas when I first came out of hospital I didn't know what was the double vision and what was the real thing . . . in the early stages I would get very frustrated because I couldn't pick up the right knife and fork or pick up a proper cup of tea. I'd go to pick up a cup of tea and I'd pick up the vision rather than the actual cup. [Now] I know what's what and what's not!

If someone has problems with their eyesight, this can affect their overall mobility. When Karen first came out of hospital, blurred vision, 'like looking through Vaseline', and double vision meant she was unable to see well enough to judge distances or heights or where the kerbs were, making it difficult for her to get out and about. Although there has been some improvement and she has been able to get back to driving, these difficulties continue to affect her life:

> I didn't realise how much my eyesight has affected me in the past year or so. It's probably affected me socially because I can only really drive for about three miles now. It's still the situation now, at just over 12 months. My vision range has increased; it's much better, but I've still got slight double vision

when I look upwards and toward my left. So when you're driving, you've got all this head turning going on and trying to get your eyes focused up is quite a strain [but] you get used to it really.

Soon after her haemorrhage Tania noticed 'a red blob kind of floating around my eyes, like a moving red dot'. Tests revealed that this was Terson's syndrome, a relatively rare condition where blood enters the eye socket and impedes vision. Having been told it might gradually disappear after 6 to 12 months, the other option was surgery. Not surprisingly, Tania found the prospect of further surgery rather 'scary' but went ahead with the operation four months after the haemorrhage so that, as she says, 'it was gone and I could move on'.

While the eyes are recovering can be a worrying period and affect, for the time being, activities such as reading and using the computer. Lesley's haemorrhage was behind her right eye, so her optic nerve was affected:

My eyes got incredibly tired . . . I'm a fast reader and I found myself having to have a piece of paper and slide it down . . . I had to do that for ages and working at the computer was just agony. My eyes became very very sore and I could do very little at a time . . . I was concerned that my eyesight might have been affected [but] it recovered as I was told it would!

So some of these problems with vision do remit over time, but the effect on people's lives can still be significant.

Epilepsy

People may have one or more fits (also called seizures or convulsions) at the time of their haemorrhage because blood is irritating the brain. This does not necessarily mean they will go on to develop epilepsy, but some do and will need long-term anticonvulsant medication (Foulkes 2004). Even if someone finds that medication successfully controls their epilepsy, it can still affect some important aspects of day-to-day life. They will not be allowed to drive until they have been fit-free for a specified period of time –

usually one year. As Vernon found, the onset of epilepsy also affected his self-confidence:

> It happened after a year; I thought I was doing okay and was rehabilitating okay and then out of the blue, all of a sudden, I had a seizure! I don't know whether it was because I was pushing myself, I was exercising at the time . . . I couldn't cope very well . . . I was like, okay, I've had the brain haemorrhage, that's one thing and now I've got to put up with this! It affected me psychologically as well. I was scared to go out too far, even outdoors, just in case something happened. I started going swimming and then I had a seizure in the pool and that made me afraid to go there again . . . But I got through that anyway, that stage of my life thank goodness [but] that part of my life I really did find hard to cope with.

Graham too developed epilepsy six months after his haemorrhagic stroke, but like Vernon he is now fit-free and able to drive again, although he regularly sees a neurophysiologist and continues using anticonvulsant medication.

Fatigue

If this part of the chapter seems disproportionately long, it is because fatigue is one of the very common after-effects. Among a group of survivors studied an average of 16 months after their haemorrhage, over two-thirds reported symptoms of fatigue (Morris 2001). Fatigue is to be expected, particularly in the very early stages of recovery. As the patient information literature points out: 'Fatigue is primarily caused by the process of brain recovery' (Kirwilliam and Sheldrick 2005: 5) and 'because your brain has to concentrate hard to process everything that is going on around you and therefore becomes tired very quickly' (Brain and Spine Foundation 2005b: 5). As Trevor Powell advises, fatigue isn't something that can be overcome by sheer willpower: 'If you've been used to driving a car with a 12-gallon petrol tank, no amount of pushing is going to make up for that lost capacity' (2004: 65). There's no shortage of advice about slowing down, taking regular breaks from activity and avoiding overstimulation.

Jarvis suggests that patients should be informed and reassured that experiencing fatigue when they get home is normal, though she also points out that research on effective ways of managing this is scanty (Jarvis 2002). Most of us think we know what it feels like to experience 'fatigue' or 'tiredness' – it's what often happens as the result of working too many hours, cramming too much into a day, not making time to relax, or not getting enough sleep, for example. But people recovering from subarachnoid haemorrhage describe their experiences rather differently:

I didn't know it was fatigue [in the early days at home]. I just felt ill, but I recognise it now. A couple of times I remember calling the doctor out, because I was so scared because my heart was pump, pump, pump. I was just totally exhausted just by doing some really simple things, but I didn't realise then that it was the sort of head injury fatigue, which is quite different. It was like no other tiredness I'd felt before and even now, I can say, well, I'm tired because I've had a late night and that's a sort of tired feeling as opposed to fatigue that is so different . . . You just can't fight it.

(Christine)

You just can't think! It's almost like a flicking of a switch really, like somebody's turning you off and unplugging you.

(Karen)

It's difficult to actually describe it; when they say 'fatigue', you just think from your past life, fatigue is tired – you've worn yourself out. You done a 15-mile trek across the cliff tops and you're shattered – but it's nothing like this fatigue.

(Rosie)

The fatigue – I've never experienced anything like that, however jet lagged I may have been in the past. To me, it's like I've done an intense time at work *and* had jet lag! It's not about sleep deprivation, it's about just being wiped out, mind numbing, no energy to do anything. And taking in information, listening, seeing bright lights, it's brain fatigue, so all your

109

functions are so wearing to you. It's exhausting just to speak
and sit with someone.

(Tania)

Others described it as their brain 'not working', or how 'the
brain aches' or the brain suddenly says 'Stop! You need to sleep
and you need to sleep now'. Certain kinds of activity could often
trigger a bout of fatigue. As Tania discovered, everyday, taken-for-
granted activities such as holding a conversation and taking in
information are tiring. Janet explained: 'I get more tired not when I
have been doing physical activities, but more when I have been
concentrating, e.g. driving, writing, using the computer.' And like
Janet, Megan found that it was 'probably the brain rather than
body fatigue, because this weekend I gardened – one day for four
hours and one day eight hours and I was fine . . . it's probably
thinking, rather than the physicalness'.

People had found different ways of managing this mental
fatigue, which could be a totally new experience. Andrew learned
to cope by understanding what was causing it and then accepting
that that's how it was:

An overwhelming tiredness, something I've never experienced
before and I didn't quite understand why that should happen; I
perhaps understand a little bit more now about how the brain
gets irritated by the mass of blood around it . . . it just seemed
strange that something like that would give you such massive
tiredness . . . You just have to go with it because there's
nothing else you can do!

Christine too recognised that this mental fatigue wasn't something
that could be overcome by sheer willpower, but initially it felt as
though she was somehow 'giving in':

You can't fight it; with tiredness you can almost pull yourself
together, keep going and you'll be all right but you can't work
through this; you have to give in to it and I think that's the
problem mentally, that you're 'giving in' to it but you have to.
Now I've recognised that, which took a while. Then I realise
that if I stop and 'give in' then I can recover quickly.

Karen sometimes found these periods of enforced inactivity quite difficult but also recognised that 'you can rest your brain and help it to heal'.

There are different ways of being able to manage this fatigue. Tania's occupational therapist helped her to tackle this in a structured way:

> She started me doing a fatigue diary, just of what activities I was doing each day and to grade the activities so that we could compare it and then she could analyse it . . . and I still keep the diaries now, because I think it was a good habit to get into.

Continuing fatigue can have a significant impact on when someone is able to resume employment. Tania delayed returning to work until she'd had a couple of months of being 'fatigue-free'.

As well as fatigue affecting when people are able to return to work, it also affects their social activities. As Patsy found, she's had to learn to sometimes say no to going out:

> I've learned to say no because there's been quite a few things, like my friends might be going to the cinema or something . . . And I'll say, 'Yes, I'm going' and then it gets to it and I'm not worried now about picking up the phone and saying, 'Look, I'm really sorry, I'm having a bit of a tough day. I'm really tired and I don't think I can do this.' And they accept it now . . . I have to pace myself.

Sometimes people found that doing things earlier in the day suited them better so they tried to schedule activities around this. For others, like Lesley, it was about slowing down and 'taking more time about everything'.

Fatigue in the first three months seems to be a universal experience as the brain is healing during this initial period of recovery, but fatigue may persist for a year or more (Foulkes 2004). This is borne out by research which found that nine months after their haemorrhage four-fifths of survivors reported continuing problems with fatigue (Powell *et al.* 2002). However, if fatigue persists, people are often able to adapt their lifestyles around it (Ogden *et al.* 1997).

Sleep disturbance

People may have difficulty sleeping at night. They may only be able to sleep for short periods, they may find it difficult to get off to sleep, or they may wake up frequently (Brain and Spine Foundation 2005b; Kirwilliam and Sheldrick 2005). Sleep disturbance can occur for a number of reasons. Problems can arise in the early stages of recovery if someone is anxious about falling ill again but without the security of being in hospital. As a result they may need to stay awake and be vigilant. As Roy described it: 'There's a fear when you come out, isn't there, that you don't want to go to sleep. When you're back home and you're in your own home, you think, well, what's going to happen? What happens if something goes wrong?' Even when he did manage to fall asleep, he would wake up again – 'probably forcing myself awake to make sure I'm okay'. Fortunately this didn't last and he can now fall asleep 'any time, anywhere I want'.

Excerpts from Veronica's diary describe her sleep disturbance in the first months after she came home:

TUESDAY 4 NOVEMBER

Had a reasonable first night but it's very nerve wracking and frightening; your imagination runs away with you. We had to set the alarm every four hours which is when I have to take my tablets.

FRIDAY 7 NOVEMBER

Had a much better night's sleep last night.

TUESDAY 11 NOVEMBER

Very poor night; seem to be getting around one hour's uninterrupted sleep. Cannot seem to get comfortable.

SATURDAY 15 NOVEMBER

Had a horrible night, troubled by dreams.

SUNDAY 16 NOVEMBER

Best night's sleep last night.

TUESDAY 25 NOVEMBER

Lousy night; very agitated and worried – woke up feeling not too bad.

FRIDAY 28 NOVEMBER

Dreadful night; thought I may end up back in hospital.

THURSDAY 4 DECEMBER

Superb night's sleep.

Veronica's sleep problems didn't last, but looking back she realises that 'a lot of it was just the anxiety' and it's not surprising that the traumatic impact of a life-threatening event affects their previous sleep patterns.

Sleep patterns can also be affected in the short term as in the early days at home people will very often have to wake up in order to take their medication every four hours, so some sleep disturbance is inevitable. As John found, getting off to sleep again at 2 am was very difficult – but night-time television was also 'dire'!

Other people's sleep problems can, however, be longer lasting. Having been someone who, he says, 'used to be able to sleep for England', Scott now uses medication to help him sleep better. BASIC (see Appendix B) has produced a booklet on managing fatigue which suggests that sleeping during the day and a lack of daytime activities can cause difficulties with sleeping at night. In the early stages of recovery, this seems to be inevitable, but if sleep disturbance persists the booklet includes some useful techniques for establishing or restoring a good sleep pattern (Kirwilliam and Sheldrick 2005: 16–18).

Headaches and head pain

Headaches are very common, particularly in the first two or three weeks when blood from the haemorrhage is irritating the brain, until it is gradually reabsorbed (Foulkes 2004). After that, headaches may continue for some time, although they are unlikely to be as severe as when the haemorrhage occurred. The literature is reassuring, pointing out that subarachnoid haemorrhage is very rare and that headaches are unlikely to be related to the haemorrhage or the subsequent surgery. Headaches can have many different causes including tension, tiredness, migraine and viral infections (Foulkes 2004; Brain and Spine Foundation 2005b). These explanations about headaches are included in the booklets for patients and carers and people may well have been told about this before leaving hospital, but have forgotten about it. Headaches are extremely common in the general population, but as the haemorrhage often started with a sudden and very severe headache, this can be a frightening reminder of a traumatic event.

When David had an 'almighty headache' at home, he was terrified that he was having another haemorrhage; although he realised afterwards that he was probably warned about this, it was a frightening experience. Fears of a recurrence are very common, in the early stages of recovery at least, often causing acute anxiety. Some survivors were having more frequent headaches than before, but others found that, despite a previous history of severe headaches, this problem had completely disappeared. Having suffered really badly with severe migraines which would last 24 hours or longer, Heather no longer has migraines at all – as she says, this is one of the only positive things to emerge.

Headaches after a brain haemorrhage can be triggered by a number of factors including tiredness, too much mental activity or dehydration. Three years after his haemorrhage, Roy's headaches have become less frequent 'but I do get headaches, mainly because it's dehydration because I don't drink very much. I should drink more . . . I had one the other day but that was because I'd been out fishing the day before and I think I got dehydrated.' Spending too long doing something which requires concentration can also be a trigger. With the help of medication from her GP, Pam has learned to manage headaches so that they don't affect her quality of life too badly:

I still get headaches, possibly very severe when I've been working at the computer. I have to take tablets and go and lie down . . . Some days it's there in the background, but it's not severe enough to impair me, to stop me doing things that I want to do anyway.

Headaches can also be the body's way of telling you to slow down. Wendy has still been unable to find a way of preventing headaches which leave her unable to work, but as she acknowledges 'it's your body's way of saying you've got to stop' so when they start, she does just that.

Several people also talked about their head pain which, they said, was not the same as headaches, although they didn't quite know how to describe it. As Rosie said:

At the beginning it was back and forth to the doctor for painkillers, because the headache . . . It's not even a headache . . . I have no faith that the person I'm telling that I have a headache has any concept of what I'm talking about, because my head hurts . . . I call it a headache, but it's not a headache like I used to have before. It's not the same . . . I'm much better now. . . but when I first came out [of hospital] I just thought I was a head; I had no concept of any other part of my body!

Taste and smell

Depending on the location of the haemorrhage, some people will find that their sense of taste and/or their sense of smell has been affected, either temporarily or more permanently (Brain and Spine Foundation 2005b). Morris (2001) found that 23 per cent of the group he studied had symptoms associated with their sense of taste, and 16 per cent said their sense of smell was affected. Jan found there were some things she could smell, but other things not at all. She couldn't smell a dirty nappy and she was also unable to smell the perfume she used – with the result that she sometimes 'overdid it'. She could, however, smell the fresh bread in the supermarket. As she says, 'It was weird', but having not mentioned this to her family, it was only when another member of her support group talked about it, that she realised others could be similarly affected.

Unusual sensations

Unusual sensations in the head are quite common, particularly in the early stages of recovery, although no one knows why they occur and they can be difficult to describe (Brain and Spine Foundation 2005b). Several people mentioned this during the interviews and all had been treated by clipping (rather than coiling), so perhaps this

115

relates to the craniotomy. Sometimes the sensations can be frightening if the experience is unexpected. When Brian developed strange pains, which he described as 'gloop inside the head', he thought, 'The clip's leaking! I can't do anything! I'm having another haemorrhage!' He was reassured that the clip was fine when he went to the support group shortly afterwards, but others have found that these unspecified sensations could easily trigger feelings of anxiety (Hop *et al.* 1998: 803). Like Brian, Veronica worried about the clip because of 'sensations in my head [when] I feel it's moving about and touching things that perhaps it shouldn't be doing'. For Patsy it's 'lots of strange noises in my head [and] creaking'. Karen-Ann described how 'my ear still creaks now. It creaks like wood, creaks inside my ear and that sometimes wakes me up!'

Janet has had 'a buzzing noise in one ear' and with Jessica's ears it's 'like being under water'. Vernon described how 'it felt as though somebody was rubbing sandpaper over the surface of my brain for a long period and I could actually feel my brain; it was a really weird odd sensation'.

Changes to physical appearance

When the haemorrhage is treated surgically by clipping, the patient's physical appearance may be altered because an area of the head will have been shaved before the operation. There will also be facial swelling, discomfort in the jaw, and pain and numbness around the scar which may be itchy or feel very cold. All these symptoms are likely to remit over time (Brain and Spine Foundation 2002; Foulkes 2004). The operation scar is usually behind the natural hairline, so once the hair has regrown the scar is no longer visible. Despite the temporary nature of these changes, people were sometimes very shocked the first time they saw themselves in a mirror. This could continue to affect their general image of themselves and their self-esteem for some time to come. Chapter 9 explores the emotional effects of subarachnoid haemorrhage.

8

COGNITIVE FUNCTIONING

Introduction

Subarachnoid haemorrhage can affect people's thinking in a number of different ways. They may have difficulties with their short- or long-term memory, concentration and attention, decision-making, taking in new information, learning new skills, and with thought processes generally (Foulkes 2004; Brain and Spine Foundation 2005b). Even when someone has made a good neurological recovery, cognitive impairments are still very common and can have a significant impact on people's lives (C.R. Scott 2006). As Shirley wrote:

> The main difference between normal pre-SAH and now is the loss in capacity of certain mental abilities. Thank heavens for technology and spellcheckers, otherwise this would probably be quite difficult to read. I find that I have to slow down when writing anything by hand, otherwise I get the letters back to front. Whereas I could do several different things at once, everything now takes much more concentration so I do find my working day quite tiring. I tend to forget things, so I make a lot of notes. I also have several 'confused' moments a day – moments where I will go into a colleague's office to ask her something and then not know what it was. People say they have these moments too but I sometimes stand up to go somewhere or do something and then everything goes blank. I can't remember what I got up to do.

Wendy also found she had cognitive difficulties and, like Shirley, they affected how she coped after returning to work:

117

> I still have days, sometimes weeks, where I feel that [my mind] is a lot slower, that I'm perhaps not taking in as much information and the response time is delayed, so whereas I might have been able to come out with some sort of quick reply . . . sometimes they have to say it to me several times and my memory is bad . . . I also feel as though I've turned into a bit of a man because I can't multitask quite so easily as I used to. So I'm doing something on the computer, the phone rings and I deal with something on the phone, [but] I can't recall very easily where I'm at on the computer. It disrupts my working pattern.

Although some people may find their cognitive difficulties persist, in other cases they lessen over time. Powell and his colleagues found that about a third of people had subtle cognitive impairments at nine months, but when they were retested at 18 months the majority scored within normal limits on most of the tests (Powell *et al.* 2004). Yet again, recovery will vary from person to person. Cognitive difficulties can indeed be 'subtle', but people are often well aware that their minds aren't working quite as well as before the haemorrhage. As Tania found:

> Cognitive testing that was done six months after [the haemorrhage] and then another six months after did highlight a disproportionate slowness in taking in visual information and then a general slowness of speed of processing information and that tied in with my experience of just feeling that I was kind of dulled down a bit in my reactions to things and needed a bit more time to read things or react. Even reacting to jokes or things that people say or ask me, I'm not so quick. Maybe I wasn't that quick before but I just feel that things are even more of an effort.

The remainder of this chapter describes people's experiences of their cognitive difficulties, discusses some specific functions including memory and concentration, and how people have learned to adapt to or minimise these difficulties.

Looking for an explanation

People often have many questions about their subarachnoid haemorrhage which can include wanting to understand the reasons for their cognitive difficulties. Did it injure my brain and in what ways? Are my problems due to the haemorrhage? Do other – 'normal' – people have these difficulties? Tania again: 'It's hard to distinguish what effect the fatigue is having on you and any actual cognitive deficits that you've been left with.' Several months after the haemorrhage, Brian was asking himself: 'That thing that you've just done wrong, is that because of some injury to your brain that happened in January or is it normal?' Plenty of people who've never had a brain haemorrhage find their memory lets them down, but conversing with colleagues doesn't stop Brian attributing his difficulties solely to the haemorrhage: 'Although he can't remember a name and I can't remember a name . . . with me it's then, I can't remember the name! I'm ill!'

People may also be unsure whether there are unrelated reasons for their cognitive difficulties such as ageing (see pp. 54–5). Fatigue will certainly affect cognitive skills and performance (Powell 2004) and people had often arranged to deal with things that required them to concentrate, for example, at those times of day when they were least fatigued.

The emotional impact of cognitive difficulties

Even if cognitive deficits are 'subtle', they may not feel so to the person experiencing them. Fear, anxiety, loss of confidence and frustration can all be triggered when they feel that their brain seems to be letting them down. Particularly in the early stages of recovery, cognitive difficulties can be very frightening. When she got home from hospital, Lauren discovered that she had to stop and work out how to make a cup of tea which, she says, 'frightened the daylights out of me'. Finding you don't know how to perform a simple task that you could previously do without thinking is scary, but anxiety can also affect cognitive performance. Tania's psychologist suggested that the results of her cognitive tests at six months could be influenced by anxiety (as well as by her fatigue).

Anxiety about whether the haemorrhage has affected the brain in some way can create a vicious circle. You start feeling very anxious, possibly panicky, about whether your brain is behaving itself, which makes it hard to think straight, so you conclude that you do have brain injury. Despite Lauren's anxiety about making a cup of tea, she was, however, aware that her intelligence was unaffected: 'I didn't have any sense that my intelligence had been damaged; I just felt my brain had been damaged.' As Hütter *et al.*

concluded: 'The post SAH-syndrome seems to resemble the cognitive deficits described after mild head injury . . . attentional deficits, disturbances of concentration and memory are prominent *without a reduction of intelligence and global intellectual functions*' (Hütter *et al.* 1995: 472; emphasis added).

Fear that the haemorrhage may have resulted in 'a reduction of intelligence' was perhaps what Brian was talking about when, soon after his return to work, he was asked to give a presentation to a group of senior colleagues – 'a huge psychological hurdle'. Brian's main concern was that 'the ideas wouldn't come out; I wouldn't be able to put my point of view across'. Prior to this he'd had a few conversations with people where he didn't think he was getting his views across or recalling the right words. In the event, the presentation went well but not without this prior anxiety. When cognitive difficulties make it difficult for someone to express themselves clearly, this can also be frustrating. As Pam explained:

> I get really angry with my husband and he's been so patient and it's because . . . if I get stuck with words or what I'm going to say, he'll [say], 'Well what *is* it you're saying? What are you trying to say? What do you mean?' And in the end I'll say, 'Well, I don't know. I don't know!' The other night he said, 'Oh what are you saying?' and I think, 'Don't! I'm not stupid – I'm stuck! Help me!'

Memory

People frequently have difficulty remembering some of their time in hospital, relying on family or friends to fill in the gaps, but ongoing problems with memory are very common. In some cases, this may only be temporary, but others may find their memory is never quite as good as it was before the haemorrhage. Long-term memory may be unaffected, so people may be able to remember events from some years ago, but frequently have short-term memory problems (Foulkes 2004; Brain and Spine Foundation 2005b). When Morris (2001) questioned people about 16 months after their haemorrhage, 70 per cent said their memory was worse than before the event. Heather has had to cope with both long- and short-term memory loss since her haemorrhage a year ago. Her long-term memories are selective – she can remember being a teenager but cannot always recall subsequent events. Her husband, Andy, can fill in these gaps and prompt her. Although her short-term memory has improved over the past few months, when her memory is unreliable this still affects her self-confidence because, she says, 'when I do remember things, I often get them wrong'. Short-term memory is often particularly bad in the early weeks or months of recovery, as Andrew found:

> Short-term memory loss was a pain . . . certainly it was bad for the first month, in that I'd have a pill and then immediately I'd forget that I'd taken the pill. I'd have a cup of tea and I'd say to my wife 'Have I had that cup of tea?' within seconds of having it.

Continuing problems with memory can also directly affect people's return to work. Seven months after his haemorrhage, David realised that this would affect his work as a chef:

> You might have six or seven things in the oven, you've got stuff on the stove cooking, and you have to send to table this and table that . . . you've got to remember everything . . . I know at the moment that I wouldn't be able to do that.

Having problems with short-term memory can be a frightening experience, as Jan found: 'I'll do something in my flat and then five minutes later, I'll have to go back because I'll have forgotten that I've done it . . . It frightens you when things like that happen, because you think you're losing your mind.' Now, however, she sees this as 'just one of those things that have happened'. Accepting that your mind doesn't work as well as it previously did is one way of being able to cope with it – a theme we return to at the end of this chapter.

Scott described himself as someone who previously had 'almost perfect recall' but now finds his memory is erratic. He has also developed confabulation – 'the inadvertent construction of an erroneous self-story' (Broks 2003: 52) – or as Scott says, there are 'some things I think I remember, that actually didn't happen . . . it's making things up and convincing myself that it has happened', though his neuropsychologist has reassured him that this is quite common.

Concentration and attention

Survivors commonly have difficulties with concentration and attention. Morris (2001) found that nearly 60 per cent of people reported that their concentration was worse than before the haemorrhage. This can affect various activities, including reading and watching television, taking part in conversations, carrying out previously straightforward tasks and doing more than one thing at a time (Powell 2004: 80–82). Tiredness, background noise and other distractions can all exacerbate difficulties with concentration and attention. Like many others, Rosie has found it difficult to concentrate, although there has gradually been some improvement:

> It's so much better now, but in the early days I couldn't even read a book. If I did read a book, I'd have to sit there with a notebook and write everything down because I was forgetting what I'd just read. Or then I'd get halfway through a chapter and think, oh, I just can't be bothered . . . I can't take in as much as I used to, but if you do it in short little bursts . . . and then do something else.

When reading was a favourite leisure activity, it may take some time before survivors are able to concentrate sufficiently to take it up again (see Chapter 11).

Distraction

Someone may decide to do something and even start doing it, but then get distracted and end up doing something completely different. When he first came home from hospital, Scott would go to the fridge to fetch a drink and come back with an ice lolly, even though he could sometimes remember he wanted a drink as he opened the fridge door.

Heather still gets easily distracted. As she explained: 'The other day when I was speaking to the lady in the flower shop where I'm going to do some voluntary work, halfway through her talking to me I was, like, "Wow, look at that flower!" and Andy was nudging me and going "Heather!"' Fortunately this means she was able to get back on track, but as she commented during our interview: 'It's very difficult keeping me on track, isn't it?'

Losing track

Many people described losing track of what they were saying – sometimes mid-sentence. During her interview, when asked about cognitive problems, Rosie explained how she sometimes gets half-way through a sentence and then forgets what she's saying, but added: 'I think I've forgotten the original question anyway!' (This wasn't uncommon during the interviews; when both interviewer and interviewee sometimes lost the thread of the conversation.)

Rosie, who describes herself as 'a chatterbox', was very frustrated when socialising in a group: 'I'd get very confused in the early days and I'd be halfway through saying something and then I found I really didn't want to continue . . . I just couldn't be bothered and I'd just stop.' Or as Pam described it: 'Between thinking something and it coming out of my mouth, it will have gone.'

Multitasking

People will often have been used to multitasking but find they are no longer able to do this. This was the case with Pam who had always been used to juggling several things simultaneously:

> I was thinking about something, while doing something else, while talking to the dogs . . . getting supper ready, talking to the dogs, thinking, oh, do I need to pick Caz up? I was thinking about my studies, thinking about work, but not now, no . . . so I don't try and do it. I focus on what I'm doing and then I don't drop things and I don't fall.

At work, as well, people are often required to multitask and it was only after she returned to work that Christine realised this would be a problem:

> I started to realise that things weren't quite right because I just couldn't do the multitasking that I could do [before]. I couldn't do the juggling and people would be saying things and I'd just forget it and I remember sitting in a meeting the first day I was back there; it was a team meeting and I just sat there thinking I haven't a clue what they were talking about. It was just going completely over my head and it wouldn't sink in, whereas I'd been used to carrying so much in my head.

Leisure activities

Previous leisure activities such as reading and watching television may be problematic after a haemorrhage when concentration is affected. People may find it more difficult to read for pleasure or that they can only watch shorter and simpler television programmes (Buchanan *et al.* 2000). We return to this in Chapter 11.

Language difficulties

Language difficulties can occur, although there is usually some degree of recovery, often in the first few weeks or months (Brain and Spine Foundation 1998). Word-finding problems are frequently reported (Morris 2001). As Kaz explained:

> Say somebody phoned, I knew who it was, but it would take a couple of seconds for me to actually come out with a name or if I wanted to watch something on the telly then I'd say 'Oh, I want to watch that programme' and I knew what it was that I wanted to watch, but it was like a delayed reaction trying to find words. I knew what I wanted to say but it wouldn't actually come out.

If someone is used to being articulate and talkative, this can be particularly frustrating. As Janice explained, having collected the author prior to being interviewed:

> As we were just coming up from the station, I couldn't think . . . 'This is a famous . . .' and the word 'landmark' wouldn't come to my mind and things like that the more you struggle to find it, the more it eludes you.

Word-finding difficulties can sometimes be unintentionally humorous. Christine is 'usually in the right vicinity of the word' but what actually comes out of her mouth will make her daughter laugh. For Wendy, mixing up her words can also produce some interesting effects:

> I either mix the words up in a sentence; it's either that or using a different word completely. So sometimes they [the family] are

quite baffled because they really don't know what I mean. Fairly recently I needed some painkillers . . . [but] said 'I need my killer pains'!

Managing cognitive difficulties

Although these difficulties are often described as being 'subtle', it would nevertheless improve people's quality of life if they were routinely offered help to manage the cognitive aspects of their recovery (C.R. Scott 2006: 36–7). Although some people are referred to neuropsychology services (see Chapter 6), several publications also include helpful practical suggestions for minimising these difficulties (Foulkes 2004; Powell 2004; Brain and Spine Foundation 2005b; Kirwilliam and Sheldrick 2005).

Survivors had often found ways of getting round their cognitive difficulties such as using Post-its or whiteboards. Others kept a diary or a list of reminders. Wendy had several 'tools' which she uses with varying degrees of success:

> I have to focus on one thing and then do another. I write things down a lot. I write lists – the only difficulty is I sometimes put the list down and then don't know where I've put it! . . . I say to people that I have a bad memory . . . so it's asking people really to just keep on nagging me and that works quite well; my colleagues at work are quite good at doing that. It's trying to use routines as well.

Skills involved in activities such as driving or finding the route from A to B are usually something we perform without having to think about it, but as Powell points out: 'Unfortunately, after a head injury some of those skills which would have gone onto automatic pilot, have to revert back to conscious thought' (2004: 81). Janice found there were things she had to relearn:

> The first time I was able to drive again, I thought, wonderful, I can go to Tesco's. I couldn't remember how you got there and this was a place I'd gone to daily for years . . . And last night I was meeting some chums at the pub I've been to in the past many times, but I couldn't remember how to get there. I had to phone and say 'How do I get there?' Of course, now I've done

it, that's relogged back into the memory. With a directional thing like that, I just ask somebody how you do it, then you do it, and follow the path they suggest and then, that is relearned . . . that's been the case with an awful lot of things.

Just as Janice had to use her brain to overcome her cognitive difficulties, Lauren also found that she was dealing with her recovery by thinking things through:

I've spent a lot of time . . . thinking through with my notepad: how do I handle this situation or how do I handle that situation? I think I'm far more cognitively aware than I was before, because you suddenly realise that you take this thing for granted that's called your brain and then it's only when it's damaged and it starts getting better you think – I can actually make better use of it than I did previously! . . . Being forced to find different ways of handling things has made me actually develop my cognitive skills to a greater extent than before.

These strategies clearly helped people address specific cognitive difficulties but sometimes it was equally helpful to accept them and refocus elsewhere. When Pam has problems with word-finding, as she says, 'I don't get stressed about it . . . oh well . . . it will come [but] if it doesn't come, it doesn't matter.' Janice has relearned some skills (see above) but she has found other ways of dealing with memory problems:

I did lose an awful lot of memory, but I think I'm coming to terms with that. I've done a lot of 'turn the page and move on' you know? Talking to myself I'd say now, you can't remember it, don't fret about it, don't struggle to try and bring it back into your mind; it will either come back or it won't . . . So that's what I've done basically and that's been very therapeutic for me.

Rosie decided that she now needed to give herself more time to rest her brain if it was going to work better:

[it] wants a bit more time to download and recharge, because my computer takes an age to download things and I feel like

we've got an affinity! And like the cordless telephone, it needs more and more charging now and it won't last as long with the battery charged . . . it was like that: you just had to spend more time recharging and less time firing on all cylinders.

9

THE EMOTIONAL IMPACT OF SUBARACHNOID HAEMORRHAGE

Introduction

Many survivors find that they feel more emotional. Recovering from a major life event and coming to terms with surviving a life-threatening illness can be a very emotionally intense time, particularly in the first few weeks and months. Mood swings, feeling low, being tearful, being anxious and lacking self-confidence can all occur, although these feelings will often lessen over time as recovery continues. The reasons for these difficult feelings aren't always clear. They may be related to the brain injury or emotional reactions to what has happened – and possibly they are caused by both of these (Foulkes 2004; Brain and Spine Foundation 2005b).

Psychological well-being may also be affected by the very sudden and enforced change in lifestyle, even if this is only temporary. Being unable to work, unable to get around in the car, and finding social and leisure activities difficult can all contribute to how someone feels. Most people will feel physically and mentally exhausted when they get home from hospital and it's not surprising if they feel emotionally drained as well. As Lesley explains:

I was exhausted and drained so I think it was more in relation to that inability to pull myself up out of that sort of sink, or pit or bog or something. And there was a sense of desolation at times, but I wouldn't have ever described it as depression. It was just I didn't have enough energy to rise out of this and I think, for me, physical and mental energy are completely intertwined so when I'm depleted physically it has that effect of causing me to feel tearful, emotional.

Particularly in the early stages of recovery it's not uncommon for people to find that their feelings are all over the place – a melting-pot of different feelings at different times. As Rosie described this:

> I'm very emotional; more so since it happened, I think. Emotions were all over the place to start with. I can remember that I was getting a different emotion every day. There was one day when there was anger, real anger that it had happened and it had spoilt everything and I can't do what I was going to do . . . And then the next day I'd be sad. And then another day I'd just feel peace. All the emotions seemed to come one at a time rather than all at once. It was almost as if someone was pressing buttons: Right! Anger today!

When people get home from hospital and begin to realise they have been through a life-threatening event, at the same time they may desperately try to leave all this behind and return to their life as it was before. When Lauren started feeling depressed and frightened, she realised 'I was trying to get back into my usual role and . . . I'd never learned . . . I didn't know how to be a patient.'

Everyone's timescales of recovery will be different and although Heather's doctors talked in terms of two to three years' recovery, after a year she is finding it difficult that things aren't 'back to normal':

> I get to the point where I'm sick of it; I just want it to be finished and over. I get just sick of everything to do with it. I just want a normal life again. I think that's probably what's pulling me away at the moment . . . And it's a realisation of what's happened. It's made such a change in your life that you didn't want.

Support services that help people when they are experiencing emotional difficulties are not always readily available, although there is increasing recognition that these problems are relatively common and need to be addressed by follow-up neurological services (Buchanan *et al.* 2000; Morris *et al.* 2004; Larner 2005). Neurosurgical follow-up is routine, but as Karen said: 'I didn't find that there was anybody looking after my mental welfare . . . I think you definitely do need some support and I could have done with a bit of counselling maybe as well.' Karen-Ann also found this was a gap in provision. She had a very supportive GP but 'at the end of the day, he didn't really deal with any of the psychological stuff; in fact, nobody's really dealt with any of the psychological stuff that happens to you after'.

Emotions may be experienced as a rag-bag of different feelings, but the remainder of this chapter seeks to place them in some sort of order, namely: anxieties and worries; feeling low and depressed; self-confidence and self-esteem; anger and frustration; issues around control, and self-blame.

Anxieties and worries

Having been through such a traumatic experience, it's hardly surprising that symptoms of anxiety are common afterwards. Indeed, they could be described as normal – a predictable reaction to an abnormal and unusual event. Of course it is possible that some people will have been prone to suffer from anxiety before their haemorrhage, but for many this will be a new experience (Morris *et al.* 2004). Feeling panicky, scared, or nervous, particularly in the early stages of recovery, is not only unpleasant but can significantly affect people's lives in terms of their return to work or participation in social activities (Morris 2001).

A recent study found that 16 months after their haemorrhage, 40 per cent of people had moderate to severe levels of anxiety (Morris *et al.* 2004), a finding confirmed by other studies (e.g. Powell *et al.* 2002). Survivors may find ways of managing their anxiety and symptoms will sometimes abate over time, but if follow-up services identified and treated it, this could substantially affect how people are able to function in their day-to-day lives (Morris *et al.* 2004).

What is it that people are so anxious about? Anxiety can be triggered for a number of different reasons. Many people are scared that they will have another haemorrhage. They may also feel anxious about returning to previous activities, such as socialising and going out, and whether they will be able to cope with other people's possible reactions to them. The fear of having another haemorrhage is particularly common in the early stages of recovery, as these experiences illustrate:

I remember being scared when I came back home; I was so scared it would happen again. And I remember not wanting to go to sleep at night in the early days at home . . . I was really scared and I'd lie down, worried that I wouldn't wake up.

(Christine)

I felt very frightened when I first came home; fears it may happen again or that I could have died. These fears subsided and only occur now and again.

(Janet)

I was happy, I was glad to be alive [but] there was still a great deal of fear; I used to be frightened to go to sleep at night . . . The anxiety was about, if I fall over and hit my head, what happens if I have another one?

(Pam)

Because headaches are very common in the early stages of recovery, even though the pain will be generally less severe than at the time of the haemorrhage, it can still feel as though history is repeating itself. As Karen-Ann explained:

It's generally the nausea that's the thing; the pain, you just think, it's just pain. If I start to feel sick, I start to get worried because that's what happened; after the pain, then I started vomiting, so it's the connection between these two and this feeling . . . urghh! But I'm not saying this is as it was before, but I'm not half as panicky now as I was because now I think if something was really hurting in my head I'd be straight down to the doctor.

Anxieties could also centre around the coils or clips (see Glossary) that were used to treat the haemorrhage. Were they securely held in place? Pam found herself wondering: 'What if this coil zips off through my brain? What if I fall down and the coil goes – phrr?' When Veronica had unusual sensations in her head, at first this made her feel anxious, despite having been told that the clip was highly unlikely to loosen:

Even now, you sometimes think, you know you've got a metal clip or a titanium clip in your brain, . . . I'm getting my confidence

131

back that I'm not going to have another bleed or that the clip isn't going to shoot off, or every time I sneeze it's not going to shoot down my nose . . . there is that thought there.

As well as these specific anxieties, there may also be more generalised fears of severe illness – as though the body can no longer be relied on to function properly; it's as if our bodies have somehow let us down. Christine went through a phase where she lost confidence. She had:

> severe anxiety about any ache or pain I had. Everything was magnified so that every spot was cancerous, every cough was some sort of serious something. Just multi-organ failures! I remember lying in bed once when [my husband] was away . . . and I knew I was about to drop dead or something . . . I would look at myself in the mirror and see all sorts of distortions that I knew were some sort of major illness . . . very rarely did I see it as another brain haemorrhage.

As Christine's experiences illustrate, anxieties can lead to thoughts spiralling almost out of control – the worst is bound to happen, the mind jumps ahead from an ache to major illness. This kind of catastrophising (Butler and Hope 1995) was also Kaz's experience after her haemorrhage:

> I was always very happy go lucky . . . [but] I'm ever so pessimistic now . . . always looking on the bad side. If anything happens, that's it! It's the end of the world which I was never like before the haemorrhage.

In many cases, anxieties will fade over time, but sometimes a vicious circle will perpetuate or worsen the panic. This is what happened to Rosie when she started feeling dizzy one morning:

> The dizziness makes you scared; you don't know what's happening. Because nobody's been able to tell you and the fear that it's bringing on makes it worse! Then you start to panic and your heart starts racing and it just makes it worse.

A reassuring visit from her GP stopped Rosie's panic. Wendy sometimes knew there was a clear reason for her anxiety, but at other times, there was no apparent reason and then, as she said, 'You get anxious about being anxious!' Vernon also realised that he was caught in a vicious circle which he needed to find a way out of:

> I worried so much about it happening again for maybe four years after . . . the more I had anxiety as well, the more I thought that it might happen again, due to the anxiety . . . So I thought, I need to do something about this, so that's when I started doing meditation.

Apart from these widely shared fears of having another haemorrhage or developing other serious illnesses, survivors' anxiety was sometimes triggered by the prospect of leaving behind the safety of their homes. Although, at first, Scott found it difficult to walk, because his difficulties weren't particularly visible to strangers getting out of the house could be a very frightening experience:

> When we were out and about, people used to try and push past me and I found that quite difficult because anything coming from behind me caused me anxiety . . . I didn't label it as anxiety at the time, but I was very anxious.

Going out also made Pam feel anxious, particularly when they moved to a new area six months after the haemorrhage:

> Initially the anxiety was about people thinking I'm drunk; okay, that's their problem; however, it's very painful to know that I'm not drunk – and I don't drink at all now . . . it was that derogatory assumption of other people that because I was slurry, because I was staggery, I was drunk . . . it was 'There's that drunk woman again. Look she's going into the "offy".' And of course I used to go into the off-licence to buy my lottery tickets!

Being at home can often feel safer and less threatening but Christine, who had been used to entertaining regularly, found this very anxiety-provoking:

133

We had a party for [her husband's] fiftieth and that's the first real entertaining I've done since [the haemorrhage]. I'd just stopped [entertaining] because it was just such a magnitude of a thing to do, plus I hated these sorts of situations where everybody's talking at once and you're trying to talk to some-body and there's somebody talking over there. I hated it; it was just awful. [And] to actually cook a meal – it was just so daunting a task. And to have everybody round and try to converse when I couldn't remember what they'd said and what had happened in their lives! You can't write everything that they're talking about, you can't keep writing it all on Post-it notes!

But how do people deal with their anxiety? Although medication is sometimes prescribed to treat anxiety, the fear or panic would gradually abate. Patsy, for example, found that 'as time goes on, I don't honestly believe I'll have another haemorrhage'. Tania described her pervasive anxieties after the haemorrhage – 'about everything in the world, my family, it happening again, if it happened to any of my family'. A neuropsychologist helped her tackle these fears, starting with a programme of relaxation exercises.

Several people talked about how, having considered their anxieties, they'd made a conscious decision to try and get on with their lives, rather than being caught up with anxieties about what might happen in the future:

At ten months [I was] realising that I could spend every hour of the day worrying about whether it's going to rebleed or realising that I could spend every hour not worrying about it. So in the end, I was just so fed up with feeling worried and it was making me miserable, I couldn't see the point to it . . . I've come to realise that if I keep thinking that way, I'm not going to be able to get on and do anything with my life.

(Karen)

I was just a bit scared that I was going to die in the night. So I decided not to go there, so I put it aside and created myself a programme of [going out and taking exercise every day].

(Lauren)

Feeling anxious about the future, worrying about what might happen, can perpetuate anxiety but Lesley found she could let go of her fears of a recurrence by not trying to control what might happen:

> Initially, there would be a different sort of feeling . . . sort of anxious . . . And now I just think, enjoy the day, make the most of life . . . anything could happen! So why stress about something that I can't do anything about anyway. Actually, in a strange and rather perverted way, I'm quite glad it happened! It allowed me and enabled me to let go of trying to control.

We return to the issue of control later in this chapter.

Depression

Feeling depressed after a brain haemorrhage is a common emotional reaction. This may be experienced as feeling generally unhappy or miserable, perhaps feeling that life is a struggle (Morris 2001). Survivors are much more likely to be depressed than if this had not happened to them, although their depression may improve over time (Powell *et al.* 2002, 2004). As with mood states generally, depression during recovery from major illness such as subarachnoid haemorrhage may either be due to the illness itself, or because people have negative thoughts about the way in which the illness has affected their lives (Larner 2005). It may also be a reaction to a life-threatening illness (Beristain *et al.* 1996). Wendy feels that her depression had more than one cause:

> I've actually been through quite a bad bout of depression which I've been told is probably linked to the bleed and the events and what's happened since then. I don't feel as good about myself, I don't feel as confident. I don't feel I'm reliable. I don't feel that I'm me. Sometimes there is a glimmer of me there, but I'm not as relaxed . . . I think depression has been one of the worst things.

As Wendy said, she also felt less confident and her image of herself was less positive; these are themes we return to later in this chapter.

Depression sometimes hits people when they get home and, having been used to round-the-clock care, they find themselves more alone. Even if they have support from family and friends, they can still feel isolated. Although fortunately Janice's depression didn't last too long, during the early stages of recovery she felt very alone:

> I felt totally isolated, very lonely, and I felt as though nobody had come to see me. I was writing down 'I've had no visitors' and this was rubbish! Loads of people were coming back and forth and I was saying 'I haven't seen a soul for three days.' Oh God, I was an absolute misery on two legs . . . I'm fat, lonely and isolated and all that sort of thing. Then it gradually got better.

Jan finally got home six months after her haemorrhage but then: 'I got rid of the 24-hour carers. I was all right for the first two or three weeks and then sort of plummeted into it . . . that's when the depression set in.'

Chronic pain can be another cause of depression. For Patsy, continuous head pain has been very difficult. As she says: 'Because I'm in so much pain all the time, I just think I don't want to do another day in pain and what is the purpose of it all . . . I did think, many a time, that I would like to have ended it all.' Despite sometimes not feeling that life was worth living, Patsy has been able to move on. She decided: 'Okay, well this has happened to me but you've still got something to give. My life will never be the same . . . but I've got a new life now – a different life!'

Although anxiety can make it difficult for people to resume previous day-to-day activities, whether it's socialising or going shopping, depression may be a consequence of people being unable to return to previous patterns of life such as going to work, driving or pursuing leisure activities (Morris *et al.* 2004). Sometimes a resumption of previous activities will not be possible. After his haemorrhagic stroke, Graham was faced with enforced retirement from work, so now he has had to find other activities which he finds can help combat depression:

> If you're feeling very low and black and depressed, as I call it, what I do is go and do something; if you're keen on gardening, go and see if you can do a bit in the garden [and] golf is my life saver.

Self-confidence and self-esteem

Survivors' self-confidence will often be affected and when they get home they can find it difficult to feel as confident as they did before the event. As adults, our self-confidence often stems from achievements that we then take for granted – whether it's holding down a job or running a home, for example. In the early stages of recovery, when these day-to-day activities just may not be possible for the time being, self-confidence may well be compromised. As a study of people with traumatic brain injury found, many of them were unsure about what they could do, now or in future, having apparently lost sight of their previous clear image of themselves (Nochi 1998). There is often a lack of confidence in daily living and in future possibilities such as returning to work. However, as recovery progresses and people are able to do more and be more independent, their self-confidence will often return. As David explained, recovery has involved rebuilding his confidence in himself:

> I was a very confident person, but since this happened . . . I look at myself and think – what? There's nothing of you! You look ill and I think because self-confidence links into your speech – definitely into my speech . . . I found that very very difficult. So if I haven't got my speech, I then become less confident. I'm getting there with my confidence, but I've just found my confidence just utterly and completely drained out of me.

Self-confidence begins to develop in infancy and during the early years of childhood as we master the basic skills such as walking, talking and eating unassisted – often with considerable pride. But in adult life we simply take for granted that our body will perform as we expect it to – until it lets us down. As Robert McCrum wrote after his haemorrhagic stroke:

> As adults we forget we live in our bodies. The unexpected failure of the body is a shocking catastrophe that threatens the flimsy edifice that we call the 'self', especially when one is reduced to the condition of a baby.
>
> (1998: 50)

The work of recovery, as Tania explained, can mean having to relearn, remaster skills which have now been lost:

You've been taken right back to the basics of learning to walk again, having your friend cut up your dinner, learning to form sounds – you've been taken back to the basics . . . you can't take for granted things that other people do. So you're cautious; I find it made me cautious about most things in life so I think that's why my confidence was so affected [and] I can't guarantee and have the confidence that when I open my mouth that it's going to come out coherently. So there's an uncertainty and an underconfidence there . . . will the shopkeeper understand me?

Self-confidence also stems from 'a model of the world, a set of assumptions' (Parkes 1998: 91). We may assume, for example, that we will get up, make breakfast, take the children to school and go to work, and that at the end of the day the family will eat together. Of course there will be blips from time to time – you oversleep or the traffic holds you up – but life is more or less predictable. As Tania found, having a brain haemorrhage upsets that assumptive world and challenges or compromises self-confidence:

I think it had a big impact on confidence . . . because when something like this happens out of the blue, it means that even though we've survived, you can't take anything for granted and you can't bank on life going ahead as you plan each day.

If self-confidence is threatened, self-esteem and self-image are also likely to be affected. The physical, cognitive and emotional difficulties after a haemorrhage, can affect key areas such as personal care, travelling, work, running the home, social life and leisure recreation – activities which often contribute to our self-esteem (C.R. Scott 2006). Nochi (1998) describes how survivors of brain injury tend 'to feel that their present selves are valueless when they compare themselves with pre-injury selves in terms of interpersonal relations, job capacities . . . and future possibilities'. Scott's experience echoes this. Having successfully set up and run his own business, he found himself unable, at first, to even handle money:

I couldn't deal with the change concept; the fear of getting it wrong . . . my own self-image was built into a lot of it. I shouldn't be having a problem with making change from a £1 coin . . . I think it stemmed from a time when I gave too much money at one point and somebody laughed at me for doing it. And those sorts of things, pre-haemorrhage, I wouldn't have bothered about, it would have been a silly little mistake but it had made a big difference because I had this whole self-image problem; I was a bumbling wreck in my mind.

So Scott felt he'd become a 'bumbling wreck', and when Karen-Ann was crying because she couldn't do something, she'd call herself 'a dozy mare'. Name-calling like this is a common example of the kind of distorted thinking which can result when self-image takes a knock. David's shattered self-confidence also affected the way he saw himself. He lost, for the time being at least, his previously positive image of himself:

I question my ability as to whether I can actually achieve something, whereas before I would never have questioned my ability, an element of doubt wouldn't have crept in . . . negativity has crept into my life which I don't like. I don't like being a negative person.

For some survivors, previous traumatic experiences meant that they had already developed skills and strategies for coping with them. Janice's husband had died very suddenly, leaving her to bring up two young children alone. As a result, she had become, she says, 'a strong and healthy woman', combining parenting with a career in nursing. But then she had the haemorrhage and '[it was] like the rug was pulled from under your feet! I hated feeling vulnerable!' Positive self-images have to be restored in recovery. Heather has also had to grapple with the loss of her previously positive self-image. Having been a wife and mother, with a successful career in advertising, now she feels 'my whole identity has been taken away . . . it's a very weird feeling and it's very upsetting'.

Even if we don't aspire to physical perfection, our self-image and self-esteem can also be affected by a changed physical appearance. Some people will leave hospital with no visible scars, particularly if they have been treated by coiling. If, however, the haemorrhage is treated surgically by craniotomy and clipping, the head will have been partially shaved before the operation (though this is often done under the hairline). Post-operative facial swelling and bruising are also common, although these may well have subsided before someone goes home.

Our image can also be about our identity. Whether or not we place any importance on our looks, the image of ourselves reflected in the mirror is what we are used to – we recognise it, it's who we are, it's us. Perhaps this is why people were sometimes very shocked by their changed appearance. As Karen-Ann said: 'I looked at myself in the mirror and that was a shock. I didn't think that thing looking back out at me was quite me.' Brian recalls his head being bandaged after surgery, but when he returned to the ward and it was removed he'd no idea what he looked like but he was, he says, 'paranoid about seeing anything'. Even after the stitches were removed he still didn't want to see himself but 'if you go to the toilet [and] open the door, there was a mirror straightway and it was a bit of a shock first time but I managed a way of getting into the toilet without looking at myself in the mirror'. Perhaps it was a case of getting used to this as Brian subsequently posted a photo of himself – complete with visible scar – on his blog.

For Rosie, her long hair was integral to her self-image, but even though she decided to take control by getting a friend to cut her hair before the surgery, she still found this difficult:

> My hair is the thing about me that is feminine. It might be bonkers but it's still this thing that makes me a girl. It took all my personality away! I wasn't me without hair! I hated it! . . . when I turned my head and there was nothing moving I hated it! And I just didn't feel it was me. I didn't look at myself until I came home anyway.

Of course, it isn't necessarily only changes to the head which people have to face. Even though weight loss and a changed body image are not uncommon, they are not always welcome. Although Karen-Ann eventually regained her lost weight, she is still not comfortable with her appearance:

> I hated it. I looked like a skeleton. I looked at myself and I was convincing myself that I looked the same [as before] . . . Sometimes now I haven't got much confidence in what I look like. I still don't particularly like looking at myself; I don't really

140

like seeing me . . . my confidence took a hell of a battering . . .
I'm a different person now.

Other physical problems can also affect self-esteem. Kaz's
operation scar was hidden by her hair, but weight loss, difficulties
with walking and an eye patch all made going out very difficult:

My self-esteem was so low when I came out . . . I just thought
all the time that people could see I had this big long scar with
big stitch marks in and because I couldn't walk properly people
would know that I had been seriously ill. And I'd be looking
round at people looking at me because I had to wear the patch
on my eye. I was just so self-conscious.

Anger and frustration

Having a brain haemorrhage can trigger angry feelings, ranging
from irritability, which is much more common, through to violence,
although the latter is much less likely. Sixteen months after a
haemorrhage, just over 50 per cent of people said they felt more
irritable than before the event, but less than 10 per cent mentioned
violence (Morris 2001). The reasons for these feelings may not be
clear. The location of the haemorrhage can affect the emotions
afterwards, but feeling angry and irritable can also be a reaction to
the trauma and the unasked for lifestyle changes or restrictions
which can ensue. Rosie recalls how angry and frustrated she felt:

There was one day when there was anger, real anger that it
had happened and it had spoilt everything and I can't do what I
was going to do . . . and 'I don't want it! Go away!' . . . and then
the frustration was, well, okay, it's happened but I can't do this
and I can't do that. The frustration probably made me try to do
more and the anger just made me want to break things.

There can be a real sense of outrage and feelings of 'it's not fair'
and 'why *me*?' As the realisation dawned about what had happened
and how her life would be affected, Heather became extremely
angry and upset:

I'd been home for a few weeks . . . and that's when I had a real 'Why me?' kind of feeling and I hadn't had that before. I hadn't been upset about it at all and suddenly I was screaming and pulling my hair and going 'Oh, why me? Why has it happened to me? Why is my life ruined?' It was strange. So yes, I have been angry about it, although I don't feel so much now, but it was just at that moment, when it all sort of came down on me.

Several people were aware that they had become less tolerant in their dealings with other people, sometimes losing their temper more frequently. Graham feels that his character has changed: 'I'm more short-tempered now. I'm not so tolerant when people say things to me.' And as Karen explained:

I think I'm probably slightly quicker tempered more than anything . . . I don't tolerate fools very well any more. I just can't seem to. I don't know, probably my patience has gone a little more. Whereas before I'd bite my tongue . . . I'd try to defuse the situation . . . now I will probably let rip, which I would probably have done years back but it would have taken me longer to let rip! Now, it's just, oh I can't be bothered to deal with this.

Finding that now you're not always quite the patient or tolerant person you were before can be difficult – as Karen-Ann described it, 'it's mouth in gear before the brain has been engaged'. She found it helpful when a neuropsychologist explained that the site of her brain haemorrhage could affect her emotions, but has still had to learn to control her angry feelings:

I was shouty, angry, stomping about the place, door slamming . . . I can still get irrationally angry, whereas before I was pretty laid back; I'm still pretty laid back now, but there is more anger in me than there was. I'm much better at controlling it now [but] in the first year I told somebody off for coming too close to me in a supermarket. I said, 'You don't understand I've had a brain haemorrhage!' I thought – 'Did you say that?'

Anger can be directed towards other people, but sometimes the survivor's anger was targeted at themselves; they were angry about the limitations imposed – even if these were only temporary. It can be incredibly frustrating to find yourself unable to perform a task which previously you did without thinking. Perhaps it feels as though your mind and body are letting you down. As Patsy explained: 'I get frustrated with the simple things like shopping, hoovering, putting clothes away, ironing.' When a friend suggested that she hadn't washed her hair very well, she recalls: 'I went into the bathroom and I was crying because I felt so frustrated. I thought, a 49-year-old woman, I can't wash my own hair! My friend's having to wash my hair! How sad is that! So I do get angry, cross.' Patsy was angry that there were things she could no longer do, but she was also having to depend on other people to do things for her. Losing your independence can be hard and we return to this issue of dependency below.

Anger and frustration often go hand in hand, particularly if, like Roy, they had always set themselves high standards: 'I've always been very harsh with myself. I want to do things right the first time, every time. [Now] it doesn't work out like that!' After his haemorrhage he has tried to be more patient with himself: 'I was perhaps a bit more forgiving of myself but I would say "Why can't I do it? Why can't I? Why can't I walk upstairs? Why can't I do it?" And I'd try again, and again and again and [then] I'd think, right, that's it – I can't! But I'll try again tomorrow.'

Among these feelings of anger and frustration there is perhaps a real sense of loss – as though the former, predictable and generally capable self is no longer present – for the time being, at least. As Wendy found:

> I get very frustrated at myself when I forget things, when I can't do things to what I think was my [level of] ability beforehand. I do find that very hard, that I'm not working at the speed I used to work at.

When someone like Karen finds themselves in tears, crying can perhaps be a way of dealing with the anger and frustration:

> I felt an awful lot of anger, I think more than anything. I suppose I would try and cope and then I'd get a day when I just couldn't cope with anything – everything was just too much and I would have tears of frustration. If I'd had a punchbag I think I'd have given it a really good kicking now and again . . . it was

just bottling things up and then I'd just have a release of it and it definitely made me feel better just to have a good cry.

In fact, Vernon did actually use a punchbag to release his anger which he found to be a helpful and healthy way of dealing with it. Scott has also found a way of dealing with his anger which at first he tended to bottle up or direct at other people:

I started going back to football and watching football. Now I've got somewhere to vent my anger and frustrations; I can shout, yell, scream, sing and do all the sorts of things there that you can't do anywhere else . . . it's an emotional venting and I think that's been quite important, going back to football.

And Rosie had inherited a good strategy which helped her deal with her anger:

My mother had this thing that she used to do when she was angry. She'd go and throw potatoes at the garden. It does help! Anything that you can get your hands on, throw it up the garden – it doesn't hurt anybody. Potatoes are good because they don't matter; they're cheap and then you can go and fetch them and cook them afterwards!

Feeling angry can be unpleasant, particularly if someone didn't see themselves as an angry person before the haemorrhage, but saying things to let unpleasant feelings escape and 'expressing negative feelings' can be helpful coping strategies (Carver 1997), particularly when they are able to find healthy ways of releasing their anger.

Dependency

While people are still in hospital, dependency on others can be accepted, tolerated, or even sometimes welcomed – it's part of being a patient. But once they get home, dependency on family and friends may not be so welcome or feel so acceptable. Having to ask for help can be difficult. There's a loss of autonomy so then you're dependent on others. Our previous image of ourselves as competent and independent adults is, for the time being at least, unavailable. Relying on other people in so many different ways can be a huge shock and it isn't always easy:

> I was more dependent on Deb [his wife] than I've ever been. I'm a very independent person; I don't need people to do things for me . . . I needed Deb to do pretty much everything: help me get in and out of the bath, help me to walk the dogs, help me put on my shoes; couldn't even lift the toilet seat . . . I just used to get angry with myself because I was incapable of doing the simplest of jobs.
>
> (David)

> I was a very independent lady and suddenly I couldn't drive a car, I couldn't walk, I couldn't walk to the end of the road. I couldn't cook a meal and I couldn't go food shopping or nip out . . . I think I'm my own worst enemy really because I try to do it all myself and I should actually ask for help more.
>
> (Patsy)

Having to use a wheelchair, even if this is only temporary, seemed to evoke very strong feelings about dependency. Graham hated this, even though it led to some unintentionally amusing scenarios:

> It's this total dependence on somebody else, because when I left rehab I couldn't walk; I was in a wheelchair, although I was damned bloody-minded to get out of the damned thing and we used to go for a walk and my wife would push me for a while and then I wanted to get out and walk. So she would walk behind me with an empty wheelchair and you would expect people to say 'Don't you think you've lost someone?'

Because subarachnoid haemorrhage commonly happens when people are in their fifties, it is likely that they will have been used to running their own lives including, perhaps, looking after a family as well. Jan had looked after her husband and five children, including three who were still at school when she was widowed, so her sudden loss of independence was hard:

> It was awful having people doing things for me . . . I think what
> angered me was because I'd brought five children up and been
> physically on the go all the time and then to be told – you've to
> sit in that wheelchair, you can't get out of it, because you've
> lost [the use of] your left side – that angers you!

Being dependent on other people also meant sometimes having to
ask for help – asking someone to do your shopping, asking someone to drive you to medical appointments, and so on. Karen-Ann
had to learn to ask for help:

> I've never asked for help before – stubborn I suppose. No I
> don't even know if it was stubborn, just independent. I thought I
> could do everything and I used to try to do everything. But I
> learned to ask; that's come to me; if I can't do something I will
> ask somebody to help me.

Lesley had been in hospital several times before, but this time she
coped with dependency rather differently:

> I had lots of experience of my behaviour in hospitals which was,
> I can do this, I can do that, don't worry about me, I'll manage!
> And this time it was just I can't manage and that letting go was
> part of this experience . . . just allow people in . . . so coming
> back and having Nick doing the cooking and things like that,
> that was great!

Like Lesley, Megan was also someone who found that being
looked after could be a positive experience: 'It's the first time I've
ever had so much done for me, I think. People were always around.
And actually in some ways it was quite nice.'

A period of enforced dependency can also have some benefits.
Someone like Lauren may be able to find a mid-point between total
independence and complete dependence. As she wrote: 'I think I
was a bit too independent before the illness and whilst I still am, I
think I have become a better team player and don't try to take too
much on board under my own steam.' Depending on others can
also mean being able to trust other people. Pam had never been
used to dependence but, as she explains, there's still that 'I'll do it

myself because if I don't do it myself, nobody else will do it right . . . but I'm better than I was.'

Control

Independence and control can go hand in hand in the sense that being independent usually means that we feel generally in control of our life. Of course, it's never possible to be totally in control (the train runs late, the cricket is rained off) but suddenly having a brain haemorrhage is obviously something over which we have no control. As the previous section of this chapter has already discussed, dependency means having to relinquish some control, but the haemorrhage itself could also be a powerful reminder that we're not always in control. As Andrew said:

> I realised we have very limited control over things in life and we don't really know what's around the corner; that's one big thing it's shown me . . . we like to think we've got control, and I'm a real control freak! And the control goes out of the window – as it did – with the brain haemorrhage.

Perhaps not being in control was one of the reasons why, soon after he was admitted to hospital, Andrew had the strange experience of thinking he was being held hostage in a prisoner of war camp. These kinds of strange dreams or memories are not unusual (see Chapter 5).

Not being able to remember what had happened immediately after they started to haemorrhage could also leave people feeling they hadn't been in control. As one of the people Jarvis interviewed told her:

> One minute I was in the bathroom and the next I was months down the road and people were telling me I'd said things to them and they had seen me and I didn't even remember. I could have died and I wouldn't have known. You think: 'Where have I been?' It was a shock to go through something and not even know and to be so out of control.
>
> (Jarvis 2002: 1434)

As discussed in Chapter 5, having no memories could be particularly difficult if they are then told that they'd behaved inappropriately (see pp. 80–1). Perhaps filling in the gaps gave them back some sense of control.

The various health-related restrictions people are advised to adhere to after leaving hospital can also raise issues of control. As Karen-Ann found: 'They said, you're not allowed to drink [and] you've got to do this, you've got to do that! All the things I wasn't allowed to do! I wasn't allowed to drive, so for me it felt like that I'd had so much taken off me.' Although clearly done with the best of intentions, being advised to restrict your alcohol intake and stop smoking (as well as having to surrender your driving licence) can feel like being taken over. Perhaps this was why some people decided to ignore the advice and resumed smoking after they left hospital? Maybe it was a bid for independence?

After the haemorrhage, as Wendy found, she needed to have at least some control over planned activities. As she explained, she needed to be certain what would be happening:

I'm not as spontaneous. If we're going on holiday I need to know where we're going, what we're going to do, where we're going to be, whereas before I could chill out about that. I get more agitated, more uptight if I don't know something's happening. Maybe it's about having a little bit of control . . . having some certainty.

If some survivors found they needed to feel more in control than usual, there was also a very positive aspect to it. As Chapter 13 illustrates, people could decide that they would take control over their recovery, by setting themselves goals, for example. As Vernon found after he got home from hospital: 'Part of me kicked in, the determined part, to say, okay, the only person who's going to do this is me . . . so I'll just do it myself, so I did!'

Blaming oneself

Hypertension and smoking are known risk factors for subarachnoid haemorrhage, but not everyone who smokes or has high blood pressure will have a brain haemorrhage. Many people will have no known risk factors and it is unlikely that they could have prevented or predicted it (Foulkes 2004; Brain and Spine Foundation 2005b). Despite this reassurance, it doesn't necessarily stop people wondering if they could have done anything to prevent the haemorrhage. With a plethora of advice in the media about 'staying healthy', people may sometimes blame themselves – at least in the early stages of recovery. However irrational the survivor's guilt may be, this may not stop them asking themselves: Was this a punishment? Have I done something bad? Did I deserve to have this happen to me? As Kaz said: 'When I came out of hospital, that's all I kept thinking – why? What have I ever done to anyone for this sort of thing to happen to me?' And as Vernon wondered:

> Was I being punished for any of the bad things and stuff that I've done in my life and this was my punishment – I went through a stage like that. But I think it's just one of those things that happen now and that is the way it is really.

Blaming oneself can also be one way of taking control, as happened when someone was told that their stroke was actually caused by genetic weakness:

> She was comforting herself by thinking she had control over the cause of her misery. Her guilt and self-blame seemed easier to bear than the thought that she was a helpless victim of a genetic weakness that had ambushed her somehow.
>
> (Raine 2000: 159)

It's a coping strategy – but not a particularly helpful one in this case. Wendy has never blamed herself because she accepted that the haemorrhage was outside her control:

> I know that it's nothing I did or didn't do; that it's not my lifestyle that caused it or the fact that I did this or didn't do that. It is beyond your control and I don't think I ever did wonder about that because I couldn't change it.

Even if someone doesn't feel they were to blame for what happened, they may still sometimes feel guilty about the impact of this on their family, friends and work colleagues. Graham's neuropsychologist helped him rationalise his guilt to some extent, but as he explained: 'There is this feeling I had of self-guilt . . . because you feel you've let your employer down, you've let your wife down, in my case I've let my daughters down.' As Tania said: 'You kind of feel guilty to see people close to you shocked and upset and worried about you', but she also wondered: 'Did I do something wrong or cause this? Why wasn't my life a bit more sorted?'

When roughly half those having a subarachnoid haemorrhage do not survive, it's hardly surprising that 'survivor guilt' can sometimes surface. Several of Megan's family, including her son, have died prematurely, and as she said:

> Sometimes I think to myself, why have I been allowed to survive? Somebody once said to me, 'You're obviously too good to die.' I said, 'That's nonsense.' [But] I've sort of got a glimmer of this feeling when [the haemorrhage] happened.

Part III

FAMILY, FRIENDS
AND WORK

10

FAMILY AND FRIENDS

Families

Although some people will be cared for by friends, or will look after themselves as 'self-carers' (Pritchard *et al.* 2001), most will be looked after by family carers – usually a spouse or partner, and in some cases by their parents or adult children. Although family carers were not interviewed for this book, survivors were asked whether and in what ways they felt family relationships had been affected.

Having a subarachnoid haemorrhage can affect many aspects of family life. Witnessing the event and being with their relative in hospital can be a frightening and distressing experience, but afterwards family members are likely to find that their own lives have changed as well. Familiar routines are probably disrupted. Personal plans (e.g. holidays) may have to be postponed or cancelled. Carers' previous employment will be affected by their new responsibilities and recreation, leisure activities and social life are all likely to change, at least for the time being and sometimes permanently. Previous studies of the psychosocial outcomes of subarachnoid haemorrhage have focused on both patients and carers (Buchanan *et al.* 2000; Pritchard *et al.* 2001) but a more recent study focused specifically on carers (Mezue *et al.* 2004).

Many of the people interviewed for this book talked about the enormous contribution their families had made in helping them to recover by providing essential practical and emotional support. As Christine had realised: 'Family is all that matters.' The overwhelming majority had relied heavily on their immediate family – partners, children and parents. For David, belonging to a close, supportive family whose members were able to share problems and support one another was invaluable during his recovery:

I think that we were close anyway, we are a close family. I believe in our family if people have got a problem that we share it. If the kids have got a problem with me, then they tell me 'Dad, I've got a problem with you' and we'll try and sort it out and vice versa. Deb [his wife] and I have always been close and the kids, but I think this has brought us even closer.

Surviving a life-threatening illness can also make people even more aware of how important it is not to take family relationships for granted. As Wendy said:

When I was in hospital it made me think, you don't know what's around the corner . . . it brings mortality home to you and makes you think, there's no point in having arguments. My mum always used to say 'Don't go to bed on an argument'; she used to dread that you may not wake up. But it does feel more true now so I'm more likely to tell my mum and dad, or my brother, when we chat over the phone, I'll just say 'Oh I love you' because I think we know that we love each other but we don't always say it.

Kaz is part of a large and supportive family and knows that without their emotional support her recovery could have been very different:

If I'd just come out of hospital and had to get on with it, then I would have sunk into a big, deep depression. But I was fortunate that I did have the love of my family and the help of them around me, because they wouldn't let me get depressed. There were too many of them around . . . they wouldn't allow it to happen. But I can imagine that it would have been a different story had I been on my own.

Tania left hospital and went to stay with her parents until she had recovered sufficiently to return to her own home. Although this might have been seen as a backward step, a loss of independence perhaps, in fact it was a bonus:

I needed family with me. And the relationships have been, although good before, ten times better. We've all talked about it and said it's almost been like a silver lining of the experience. I've got much closer to my parents; really I would say they're now my friends – and my brother as well, we've grown much closer . . . in some ways, my friends and family, they really made my recovery for me so I feel very lucky.

But not everyone will feel as lucky. Traumatic events can bring families closer together and strengthen everyone, but if there were tensions and difficulties before the event, it may be more difficult for everyone to come together and offer the emotional and practical support people need to help them recover. Sometimes other family members are unable to cope with the newly dependent person. In Pam's family, she'd always been the one who looked after everyone else but now:

There seems to be a bit of competition about. 'How come you've got a disabled sticker for your car? At least you can drive! . . . And how come you get disability living allowance?' . . . I'm no longer the one in the caring role . . . I wasn't there for them.

It is also important to point out that some people may have few or no family members to turn to in recovery and have had to find alternative sources of support – turning to friends, perhaps, or relying on their own resourcefulness in order to make a successful recovery. The role of friends is discussed below.

Spouses and partners

The trauma for someone witnessing their spouse or partner collapsing or being given the news that they are critically ill and have been rushed to hospital cannot be underestimated. After their relative comes home from hospital 'some partners were afraid to leave the patient alone, especially if they had witnessed the traumatic event' (Hop *et al.* 1998: 803). It was only 18 months later that Shirley became aware of how the ordeal had taken its toll on her husband. As she wrote:

I was unaware that, for some time, he has been having panic attacks and the stress has made him quite ill. It came to the point where he was taken to hospital with a suspected heart attack. Thankfully it was not. It was only then was he asked if he had spoken to anyone about the whole thing – he hadn't. He wasn't even aware there was anyone he could talk to.

It was only after his suspected heart attack that they were able to start talking together about what had happened and he could begin to recover from the experience:

He was so apologetic because he felt, as men do, that nothing had happened to him and he should be stronger and able to deal with it. In his words, 'It's all in my head and if I feel like this, how on earth must you be feeling!' He had been loathe to talk to me about the SAH in case it upset me. I have explained that I was blissfully unaware of most of the ordeal. I didn't have to watch my partner collapse and have fits. And thankfully I didn't have to wait outside the operating theatre for seven and a half hours. How could it be so much worse for me? . . . The tablets he was prescribed have gone into the bin. His headaches have stopped completely and the rash has nearly gone . . . He says he feels absolutely great now.

In Wendy's case, it was when they went for family therapy (because their daughter had difficulty leaving her mother and going to school) that her husband was able to talk about how frightened he'd been when the haemorrhage occurred. This enabled them to talk about the impact of her sudden collapse:

So now he's a changed man and we talk about our feelings a lot, about what happened . . . I think we've got a much better understanding of each other. We've been married almost 25 years and I think now we're closer than when we first got married . . . So it's been really good in that respect.

When one half of a couple has a serious illness such as a brain haemorrhage it can be the catalyst for a number of changes – from carer to patient, for example, from main or sole breadwinner to being unable to work (Ogden 2000: 57). They may be unable, for a time at least, to parent their children or run the household. A husband or wife may no longer be able to contribute to the family income. Heather had combined several roles – holding down a demanding job, running the house and looking after their son. After the haemorrhage it was 'definitely role reversal'. Having previously done the shopping, cooking, cleaning, tidying and washing, her husband had to take it all on – as well as looking after their young son. As she found, 'suddenly you feel like you're about twelve again'.

People were often aware of the stress resulting from these enforced and unplanned changes. Although Patsy has gradually been able to do more around the household, she still needs her husband's help which has to be fitted in around the demands of his job:

> because he does more around the house perhaps than he used to do. I find I go to the supermarket and he meets me there because I can't do [the checkout and packing] but he usually finds me in the aisle going 'Oh don't leave me where I am!' so I think I have put an extra strain on him because he works hard, works very long hours and I used to do a lot of gardening and I can't do that so well now.

If someone has been used to running the household for many years and doing it in their own way, it can be quite difficult when their 'other half' has to take over. In the past Karen's husband's job often took him away from home for long periods, while she ran what she describes as 'quite a chaotic house' and looked after their children. The switch of roles when she came home from hospital wasn't easy:

> Obviously he was always used to me being there and doing everything I suppose and . . . he likes to be in control; he likes everything to be just so. He liked to be on top of everything and it was sort of done to military precision when I came out! . . . Everything was sort of timetabled and I found everything so unrelaxed . . . it was just very strange; it didn't feel the same.

Relying on the other person to help with household tasks means being able to ask for and accept that help, but as Carleen Scott's study found, with close relationships this actually improved their quality of life (2006: 38). Wendy still finds it difficult sometimes to relinquish what she sees as 'her' jobs, but is still glad of her husband's help:

> Before the haemorrhage I was a very busy person. My husband was out working long hours so I would run the house and look after my daughter . . . I'd be the person running round after everybody else and then suddenly the tables were turned . . . My husband had to take over doing all the household tasks . . . so he's learned to wash, learned to iron, he's learning to cook and part of me feels really glad he does that much when there are times when I just don't want to be bothered with it. And there are other times that it really gets me down because I'm thinking that they're my jobs and I should be doing them.

When someone gets home from hospital their 'patient' status is likely to continue for some time, but as recovery continues the often delicate balance of the carer/cared-for relationship may need to be renegotiated so that it becomes, or returns to, being more interdependent and perhaps less protective on the carer's part. As Graham says, 'there is a huge difference because she's not just my wife, she becomes my carer', which can strain their relationship:

> My wife has been so caring for me all our married life, but over the last nine years [since the haemorrhage] it's difficult for her now to switch off and let that bit of rope go a little bit further. She's overprotective with me still . . . and it's difficult for her to switch that off.

Whether this is 'overprotectiveness' or understandable anxiety, partners or spouses may still continue to worry. James has absolutely no worries about having a haemorrhage, but that doesn't stop his wife worrying sometimes. Karen-Ann knows that if she gets a headache or a pain her partner, Mark, still worries, though he won't voice his concern.

It is not unusual for people to want to go out less after their haemorrhage (an issue we return to in the next chapter), but this can lead to changes in a couple's previous lifestyle. Scott has not yet been able to return to work and prefers to spend more time at home, but he also recognises that his wife's life has changed too:

The whole event has changed everybody's life around me. Sarah, pre-haemorrhage, used to be at home with the kids all the time. I used to get fed up with her going out for a meeting even if it was just one a week . . . Sarah now has an outside life; she's got a wide group of friends now . . . she's a lot more independent than she has ever been . . . whereas I've become a lot more socially withdrawn than I was.

Because Graham has been unable to return to work, he and his wife also had to face life in retirement but, as he points out, 'With normal retirement, you can plan it – this you can't! You're chucked in and that's it.' However, they have found ways of managing their time by having both shared and separate activities. Graham plays golf with friends and 'it gives her space and it gives me space which is very vital in a relationship'. They also have one day a week 'where my wife and I can spend some time together, because it's important that we do, for our relationship . . . sometimes you can talk through a problem when you're walking'.

One or both partners may be nervous about resuming sexual activity, particularly if the haemorrhage occurred while having sex (Hop *et al.* 1998). Although libido may be somewhat lower (Buchanan *et al.* 2000), the advice is reassuring: 'Sex presents no risks' (Brain and Spine Foundation 2005b: 7); 'It's safe to have sexual intercourse as soon as you feel ready' (Foulkes 2004: 33). Andrew's haemorrhage occurred immediately after intercourse, but the next time it was his memory that almost got in the way:

This was obviously something we had to overcome and we both needed to face up to that . . . because otherwise it would mean we would never have sex again . . but the strange thing is, we did have sex and I forgot about it and I said to my wife 'Did we have sex?' And she said, 'You know we did!' I said, 'Did we?' And it was really strange because I'd almost forgotten. But I'm still here to tell the tale.

Veronica's haemorrhage started while she was in the gym but, like Andrew, there was still some apprehension:

In the early days I read in one of the pamphlets I've got here that . . . one of the most likely times to have a subarachnoid brain haemorrhage is during intercourse! So of course . . . you're really very, very scared initially. But if you've got a caring partner . . . things are now back to normal and that's no problem.

Despite the strain on relationships which can occur, people also recognised the positive effect that this had had. As Janet wrote: 'I feel it has brought my husband and myself closer.' And although Rosie and her husband had had some difficulties in the past, she sees how her haemorrhage has enriched their marriage:

It drew us really close together, closer than we've ever been. So it was good, it was almost like we could start again . . . And it shook us both up and shook us into ignoring the trivia and looking at what's really important.

Roy and his wife had only been married for two years but he now feels this has brought them even closer together and that they have both benefited from the experience:

Since then we've got closer and I think as every single day goes on, we get closer – even now. I think because we've got a 'history' behind us now, so we share that and as every day goes by that improves, that history grows, becomes more enriched. I think Joan became more tolerant of my failings, which had a mirror effect on myself. I became more tolerant of her failings!

Although there may be deepening relationships for some couples, others may have decided during their recovery to make a new start and leave their marriage behind, although they would not necessarily attribute this to the haemorrhage. As Vernon acknowledges: 'It had a bit of an impact on our divorce but I think it was sort of coming anyway . . . then the brain haemorrhage happened so I think that was a separate issue.' After her second haemorrhage, Sandra was clear that deciding to separate from her husband could not be postponed indefinitely:

I'd known for a long time that I was very unhappy. And so it gave me the courage because I knew that only 'now' matters. I couldn't keep putting it off any more. I kept saying, well, I'll wait until the children are older – and then one day I thought, well, how old have kids got to be? . . . in the end I couldn't deny that I had to deal with it now. I'd given it a lot of thought and it wasn't a whim; it was a serious decision.

Children

Children of all ages will be affected in one way or another. They may have seen their parent collapse and be taken to hospital, but even if they were not present they are still likely to have visited them in hospital, perhaps seeing a gravely ill mother or father unconscious and surrounded with all the paraphernalia of an intensive care or high dependency unit. The other parent may have to decide how to explain what has happened and how much information to give them. Andrew's six-year-old daughter was at home on the morning when he collapsed and saw her father being taken to hospital. Since then, they have talked with her about what happened:

> She cried after I went and it's obviously quite traumatic to see your dad go out and get carried away and not [be] sure what's going to happen to him. It was quite frightening for her . . . but I actually think she came to terms with things quite well; she had her mother there; and we do still talk about it. I say to her, 'Do you remember the time when I saw your picture of the ambulance?' 'Oh yeah,' she'll say, 'I did that because that's the last thing I remember as you went out of the door.' She said she was scared coming into the hospital but then she'll go off and say 'Oh, I went round to Aunty Ros's.'

Andrew's daughter drew a picture of the ambulance which took her father away and she was also able to talk about what had happened. Reconstructing the story of a traumatic event like this can be helpful (Herman 1994). At first Karen's teenage daughter needed to talk again and again about what had happened, although this eventually faded:

> Lauren spoke endlessly about me having the haemorrhage . . .
> It probably did go on for about four months and she was

> forever saying 'Oh Mum, do you remember this and remember that?' and, yes, very emotional, very emotional . . . she'll still talk about certain aspects of it, but before it seemed to dominate the conversation, that's all we had to talk about. Obviously she must have needed to talk about it . . . and it's finally petered out.

It is not only the survivor who worries about another haemorrhage. At first, Karen's daughter was also not keen on going out and leaving her mother at home. Similarly, Wendy's six-year-old daughter went through a phase of not wanting to go to school in case she came home and found her mother had died. Children of all ages can be rather protective but older children can provide practical and emotional support as well. When Megan was first home from hospital, for example, her daughter would visit every day after work as well as taking her mother shopping from time to time.

Parents also noticed that, as their recovery progressed, their children would often revert to their previous patterns of relating (which is probably very healthy for all concerned). Janice had been widowed for some years when she had a second haemorrhage and though her grown-up children were initially protective and supportive, as she says: 'This is wearing off now – "She's all right now! Move on!".' Similarly, Patsy found that 'they were absolutely brilliant when it happened, but I think as time goes by, it's the same old story, they look at me and I'm mum, aren't I?'

Perhaps it can be helpful to feel that your 'temporarily suspended' parental role has been handed back to you by the children? During their parent's recovery, children are also getting on with the business of growing up. As Wendy says, although at first her daughter would tell her mother to sit down if she saw she was tired: 'This doesn't happen very often now. She's a normal teenager now.' After his haemorrhage David realised that children's – quite reasonable – assumption that their parents are there to look after them no longer works in quite the same way, for the time being at least:

> The parents are always there for the kids and the kids usually fall over and they're ill. The parents aren't generally ill but it shows the kids that your parents can be ill, we're only human . . . I think it has opened all our eyes up.

162

When a parent is recovering at home, one of the potential benefits is being able to spend more time with the children. Scott feels that, as a result, he and his sons now have a closer relationship. He's also become more involved with the boys' school and his older son has used his dad's MRI scan as a project to showing the brain as a 3D model. Parent and child can both benefit from this shared time – and for Wendy it also helped her recovery:

> One of the best things was my daughter was doing her SATS [school tests] and because I was off work, I had time to sit with her and go through her maths with her. I could cope with about 20 minutes of mental maths . . . so that was something really good that came out of me being poorly.

Friends

When someone hears that one of their friends has had a brain haemorrhage., it's likely that this will be something they've never encountered before. They may have visited their friend in hospital, who might still be very ill, or they might go on to the ward and see someone who doesn't appear to them to look very different (particularly if the haemorrhage has been treated by coiling). Friends can find the prospect of hospital visiting very daunting. They may be frightened about what they will see and what their friend will be like:

> I remember a friend coming . . . and she said to me 'I was frightened to see you!' and I think that's what a lot of people are . . . I don't know what they expect . . . I think people expected me to have two heads!
>
> (Patsy)

> I think people think 'brain' and of course, if it's a close friend, if it's somebody you care about 'Do I want to see my close friend altered? Am I going to see an imbecile in the bed?'
>
> (Pam)

Friends' awkwardness can stem from having no clear idea of the possible effects of a brain haemorrhage and from fears that they

163

won't know what to say or whether the other person will be able to communicate. As Rosie explained:

> They think you're going to be a different person or lost your marbles; they think perhaps you're going to be a bit mentally inhibited and that they're not going to be able to talk to you; they're not going to know how to deal with you.

Of course, if someone has speech difficulties then conversation can be awkward, as Pam found after she came home from hospital. Despite the fact that her friends were the nurses and doctors she'd worked with:

> They became tongue tied. People would come round and visit . . . but because I couldn't communicate properly at that time, they just didn't know how to be with me. And they were upset as well and very slowly they all dwindled.

Even without speech difficulties, conversations with friends can still be awkward. Karen-Ann described how a friend visited her in hospital and 'her lip was definitely stuck to her teeth'. Eventually, she concluded, there is this awkwardness 'because people don't understand what's happened and they can't think of anything else to say so I don't think there's any malice in it'.

Individuals can react very differently to illness or injury. As Karen said: 'People react to it differently, I suppose, depending on what their character was like in the first place.' Some may take it in their stride and be seemingly unfazed. Others may find the whole idea of brain injury very threatening. Friends sometimes react in unexpected ways. Some will cope better than others and, as often happens with a bereavement, some friends will be more comfortable with offering practical help, while others will be able to offer a listening ear:

> It's extraordinary – people that I thought were my close friends sidled away and other friends that I'd sort of lost touch with were all crawling out of the woodwork, suddenly appearing . . . Two of them came rushing up to me in hospital saying 'Oh, we're so sorry we've not been in touch properly and let's put a stop to that!' I've regained a lot of friends that I thought I wouldn't see again.
>
> (Rosie)

I found that people fell into two categories. There were people who just had a natural empathy and were just able to take one look at me and say 'Do everything at your own pace' and were gentle with me. And there were others that were impatient and couldn't understand it.

(Lauren)

When something like this happens to you, you really find out who your friends are. We've got two very very good friends – the best friends you could ever want . . . absolutely fantastic. And friends we thought were good friends sort of cold-shouldered you a bit . . . they wouldn't want to know how you were progressing . . . I don't know whether because they knew I'd had brain surgery, whether their mental picture of someone with brain surgery would be, you know, he's going to have a big bandage on his head and he's going to have tubes coming in and out of him left, right and centre.

(David)

As these comments illustrate, survivors generally accepted that friends' reactions to the haemorrhage and the way they coped with it weren't always going to be predictable or consistent.

Because brain injury can be largely invisible, friends may find it hard to understand what has actually happened and what the possible effects of a brain haemorrhage are likely to be. As Patsy commented: 'I just think people don't understand how the brain works.' And as Karen-Ann realised, if you're still struggling to understand what's happened and how it's likely to affect you, it's not going to be easy to try and explain this to friends:

because I couldn't tell them, because I didn't understand what had happened myself. Some perhaps understood how much more serious it was than others; other people saw Karen-Ann being who Karen-Ann was so nothing really bad could have happened to her . . . I don't think they realise that if you're haemorrhaging inside your brain it's a very dangerous place to have a haemorrhage because it's the damage that's done. I don't think that people generally realise that.

When someone has made a 'good' neurological recovery but has some difficulties, friends may not always be aware of these 'hidden' problems. As Rosie found, friends wanting her to socialise didn't always understand her fatigue:

> They'll look at your calendar on the wall and they'll say, 'Look, you've got two days there.'
> 'Yes, but I need "me" time.'
> Most people understand but some people don't: 'Oh well, you could do that.'
> 'No, because I will be exhausted.'
> 'Oh well, we all get tired.'
> 'Well, no, not like this!'

However, Rosie did find it useful to show a friend a booklet about subarachnoid haemorrhage – 'and my friend pounced on it and avidly read it because she wants to understand. She still doesn't entirely understand but she's trying to learn and she's keen to know.'

'Subtle' cognitive difficulties can feel anything but subtle. Pam found it hurtful when people sometimes expected her to be the same person she was before her haemorrhagic stroke:

> Unless it's happened to anybody, I don't think they can understand the blankness, or perhaps I have been more eloquent in the past and now that isn't so! . . . they've said 'You're not stupid, so what's going on with you?' That is when I get angry.

Roy also found it hard to explain to friends how the haemorrhage had affected him. Although friends were generally sympathetic, he felt there was a lack of empathy – they couldn't really understand what he was going through:

> They sympathise with you – 'Oh, sorry to hear about that' – but they don't seem to be able to get down to the level that you feel yourself inside and that's perfectly understandable. It hasn't happened to them, so why should they? . . . They don't feel what you're feeling.

Most people don't particularly like it when things change. If a good friend isn't exactly the same person we've always known, the struggle to recover may not always be acknowledged. As Graham found, although he has worked hard to recover, friends are sometimes unwilling to acknowledge his continuing difficulties:

> Some of my friends have known me for 30 years and they know that I've had a brain haemorrhage and a stroke [and] subsequently epilepsy, and it's taken me nine years to get to the stage I'm at. And they turn round and say, 'There's nothing the matter with you, Graham!' and I say, 'Well, you obviously don't know me very well to make a statement like that!'

Recovering from brain haemorrhage often takes considerably longer than survivors themselves expected and the same can go for friends. Perhaps this isn't surprising. If a good friend has been ill, then we probably want them to recover as quickly as possible – we want our old friend back straightaway (why else do so many cards have the message 'Get well soon!'). As Tania found, when her speech had begun to improve and outwardly she seemed better:

> It was evident in the early days that I was very tired and exhausted and . . . when I had the eye operation . . . everyone was very fine about that and just said 'Well, we can't know how you feel' because I didn't look as bad as I was feeling, but they were accepting of whatever I said. But after, say, six months or seven I started to kind of branch out and do some more activities. I looked okay and my speech had really started to recover and so I think it was hard for some people to really understand that I was still going through the emotional recovery . . . [and] because they could understand [her speech], they couldn't really understand why it was a problem for me.

As Rosie too realised, other people can find it hard to take on board that recovery is long term, but deciding how to respond can also be difficult:

> Most of us have never had anything worse than flu before . . . but you're over that in a matter of weeks; people cannot comprehend that an illness can take you such a long time to get over. They don't want to comprehend. Quite a lot of people say

167

'Are you 100 per cent recovered?' and you say 'No, not quite', and then you think, oh that was the wrong answer because they don't want to know that!

There's a delicate balance to be struck between letting friends know what you're going through or keeping things to yourself. Patsy decided that even though she might not be feeling too good she'd rather not let friends know that:

> They look at me and they think 'Oh, she looks okay now'. And because I try and do all these things, they think I'm all right . . . and I don't let people see me at my worst, I suppose . . . they don't catch me crying or whatever.

As the final chapter of this book explores, having a brain haemorrhage can be a life-changing experience – and often a very positive one – but these changes may not always go down too well with friends. Pam feels that some aspects of her personality have changed:

> I think [the haemorrhage] has altered mine in the respect that I'm a lot more positive now. I will get up and go . . . I've got a horse and sometimes it will take me four hours to muck out each day, whereas some days it'll take an hour because I'm okay. But I'll do it and I'll stick to it and I think I'm a lot more determined, but some don't like that either.

Patsy has also realised that her friends can find it hard to accept that she cannot always do things as before:

> I think whereas before I was at everyone's beck and call but if they picked the phone up, I will say 'I can't do that now' and it's hurtful sometimes to think that people look at you differently. They don't want me – this new person!

So there can be difficulties and misunderstandings and sometimes friendships may have to go through a period of mutual adjustment, but despite all this many survivors are also well aware of how friends have supported and encouraged them during their recovery. As Graham found with fellow golfer Mike:

I've not known him that long really, but he is very caring towards me. He'll say, 'Look, if you're not up to it, we'll pack up after this hole.' And I'll get back to the car and we're putting all our gear away and he will put all my gear in the car for me – just simple things like that, just to help . . . Really, in a way, it's quite a tender thing, coming from a bloke that's six foot five. You wouldn't expect it.

When people were still in hospital they sometimes found that people they hadn't been in touch with for years were at their bedside and friendships that had withered away were rekindled. Sandra knows that some people didn't visit her because they were too scared: 'But by the same token, I never knew I had so many friends! People that just appeared from years ago – and cards. Just so many good wishes!'

Sometimes support came from unexpected quarters. As Scott had to accept that his life would never go back to how it was before:

It was the strangest people in the world that have accepted that – acquaintances, people I'd have associated as being Jack-the-lad before my haemorrhage have been far more under-standing in certain instances than people I would have thought of as sensitive and caring.

11

SOCIAL LIFE AND LEISURE ACTIVITIES

Introduction

In the early weeks and months of recovery, particularly if people had previously worked full time, they are likely to find themselves with a great deal more 'free' time. At first they will probably need to get plenty of rest, but leisure and social activities can also play an important part in recovery. Participating in a range of activities can help people maintain their social relationships and generally enhance their quality of life (C.R. Scott 2006). The extent to which people can resume previous leisure and social activities will, of course, depend on the extent of any disabilities they have sustained as a result of the haemorrhage, but if someone is less active than before, this may also be because they have made the positive choice to adopt a different lifestyle (Powell *et al.* 2004).

This chapter explores the ways in which people's patterns of socialising were affected, their experiences of going out, the impact of possible restrictions on driving, and their participation in sports and exercise and home-based leisure activities such as reading and watching television.

Socialising

People's previous social life can be affected by a haemorrhage for a number of different reasons. Cognitive difficulties, feeling very fatigued, not being allowed to drive, finding it difficult to tolerate a noisy and crowded environment can all mean that, for the time being at least, people may find socialising difficult (Foulkes 2004; Brain and Spine Foundation 2005b). At first Christine did not always want to spend time with other people, but socialising is gradually becoming easier, although entertaining and talking with friends can still be difficult and tiring at times:

Relationships with friends took a dip . . . I did withdraw from society for a while, but we've rekindled quite a few groups of friends . . . there was definitely almost a tongue-tiedness, I suppose. I find that I can find myself slowing down even now. I've always loved to talk and I could talk for England but I find that talking is really the hardest thing, that knocks me out.

Patsy too finds socialising hard work but also recognises the effect this has had on the rest of her family. Social activities, particularly sometimes deciding to do something spontaneously, can no longer be taken for granted. Now she has learned to plan and pace herself to take account of continuing fatigue:

I find if I wanted to go out this evening, for example, I'll do nothing all day, whereas before . . . I'd nip here and there, so I find, socially I can't do it. I get so so tired . . . But I also feel it affects my family too, because they're not the ones who are not well, but their lives have had to change too, to adapt to me . . . I've had friends here all weekend and that's worn me out completely, but even having people for a meal or something is hard; everything is hard work now . . . things we took for granted before.

Fatigue can often be unpredictable which makes forward planning of social activities difficult. Because Karen can only drive short distances, friends mostly come to her house, but even so she sometimes has to cancel at the last minute:

There have been many times when I've had friends coming over for a coffee and I've had to cancel them because I've felt just too tired. I probably thought, if I'm tired, I can't make conversation because I can't think straight and they'll get bored witless, sat with me.

For someone like Rosie, who describes herself as having been 'a party animal', she – and those around her – have had to get used to the way her social life has changed:

I was always out at parties, up the pub, life and soul they used to call me . . . We had a party at a friend's beach hut last weekend and they were all expecting me to be the last one to leave and I was drinking ginger beer and went home early!

For reasons that aren't altogether clear, Pam found that, at least in the early stages of recovery, her sense of humour seemed to have disappeared and she was unable to follow the jokes and banter which can often characterise social occasions:

I didn't really know what people were talking about and I didn't know what was funny and what wasn't funny. . . so it was about joining in conversations . . . things were too fast for me. I couldn't keep up. 'What's funny about that?' It would be explained to me and then the power of the joke would have gone.

People also found that they were often drinking less on social occasions. Drinking alcohol 'in moderation' is okay (unless contraindicated because of medication) but people may find that they feel drunk or become sleepy more easily than before (Brain and Spine Foundation 2002; Foulkes 2004). For Vernon, the haemorrhage has changed his drinking and his patterns of socialising:

I do go to the pub, but not as often as I would have done before. And drinking – I'd like to just not bother to drink. I was just thinking recently . . . well, I don't think I'll bother drinking at all now because I've been out several times with [his partner] and not bothered drinking and I've enjoyed it more because I can remember all the evening as well! . . . I'm more affected by drinking since the haemorrhage . . . I'm probably not quite as sociable as I used to be . . . I've got several close friends and I think I'm quite happy with that.

It seems to be quite common for people to find that they now prefer being in a small group of friends, rather than participating in larger social gatherings, particularly if they are likely to be noisy (Buchanan et al. 2000). As recovery progresses they may feel more confident about being in larger groups, but as Tania found:

I've been very cautious about social things and until very recently I've only been able to cope with no more than two

172

people at a time and not inclined to go to any big parties . . . I just really only want my close friends. At first I didn't go to any social things for at least six months and the first one was just . . . a little gathering . . . I'm a little better now . . . but I do find socially I'm not interested in anything that's bigger or more loud. I don't want to go to any loud bars or clubs.

Scott is someone who also goes out much less than before, but he still finds socialising very tiring and is unsure whether friends who know him well really understand how the haemorrhage continues to affect him. As a consequence he is less keen on going out:

I don't feel the need to go out as I used to; I don't mind going round to other people's houses, because it's a smaller group. Because I tend to try and do a lot I tend to get tired and I haven't found the right balance yet . . . tonight [after the interview] I'm just going to veg out in front of the TV . . . even the people who know me well don't understand what all this means to me. We shouldn't care what other people think, but I always feel that people expect more of me . . . I'm not going to withdraw completely socially, but it's not something that I have a great urge to do any more.

In this and the previous chapter, people were often having to renegotiate friendships, but what about meeting new people who may know nothing about the haemorrhage? Do you even mention it if you appear 'normal'? And if you do, what do you tell people? Pam moved to a new area soon after her haemorrhage and when she goes horse riding, she does mention it, not least because she feels that saying nothing would be irresponsible: 'If they're out with me and I perhaps fall off and bang my head and I'm dead.' Lesley also had to tell people she hadn't met before when she started psychotherapy training very soon after her haemorrhage:

I remember walking at what felt like a snail's pace into the room and hardly even being able to carry my bag . . . and we did our round of introductions and I said, 'If I'm a bit out of it, this is the reason.'

173

Lesley was obviously still unwell when she had to meet a roomful of strangers but where someone's disability is perhaps not so obvious to other people, it's less easy to decide whether to say anything. As Tania found with her speech difficulties:

> I'm torn as to whether to have to apologise for it to people, to say upfront 'You'll have to excuse me; I've had a stroke and my speech is a bit ropy' . . . or just plough on and pretend that nothing is wrong because a lot of people try to make me feel a bit better and say that they don't hear anything. And I think that's because they're either not paying attention or they're just being polite. But if that is true, then it would be crazy to start speaking up and talking about a problem that people don't even notice!

Going out

Going outside the home can be difficult, particularly in the early weeks of recovery. As the previous section of this chapter discussed, it can not only affect people's social life but also other activities previously taken for granted – shopping, exercising the dog, going for a walk, swimming, or going to the gym, for example. Even though he'd been warned that going into crowded and noisy places was likely to be difficult at first, Andrew's first outing, a few weeks after leaving hospital, was an unnerving experience:

> I remember it was near Christmas. I went to get a present for my wife, with my sister; she took me in her car . . . going out into a crowd, I felt terrified! The first time I went out, it was just horrible, I felt a real fear. I felt vulnerable. I'd lost my confidence.

A combination of physical and/or sensory disabilities can mean that even a previously simple task like shopping can be rather fraught. As Karen found, problems with her eyesight and being surrounded by different noises was difficult when she ventured into her local supermarket. There were:

> crowds of people and you're thinking about what to buy and you're looking for something, your eyes are all over the place

and you can't see very well. [There was] piped music, and one time there was a security alarm going off at the door as well.

Perhaps particularly when someone has had a craniotomy, their head can feel very vulnerable. Karen-Ann remembers going to the supermarket and using a trolley as a barrier to protect herself:

> It was terrible! I hated it . . . the shelves were so high, the boxes balancing precariously according to my view of the world at that point! [They] might fall on my head! The trolley always went to the right of me and I'd rather run people over with the trolley than have them near me . . . if someone comes too close, I'll get them with my trolley. And I'd hold on to the trolley like that was my lifeline.

She also found the prospect of going to the hairdresser another frightening experience:

> The first time I went to the hairdresser – what a palaver! . . . I wasn't willing for them to wash my hair; I didn't really want them touching my head . . . but they were brilliant! My hairdresser who I've gone back to ever since [the haemorrhage] is brilliant . . . she was so gentle. They've looked after my hair ever since and I wouldn't go to another hairdresser because I'd have to explain to them what had happened.

After her second haemorrhage, when the hairdresser's scissors accidentally touched the site of the craniotomy, Sandra decided to do her own hair in future but, like Karen-Ann, she was still worried that someone would accidentally knock her head:

> I couldn't sit on a right-hand corner; I couldn't expose my head to the right side because if I was sitting, my head was at someone's elbow height and I was always conscious that if someone was walking by and they'd turned round, that part of my head was exposed to danger . . . your head is so exposed! I became very very paranoid . . . my left side you could hit with sticks – I don't care what you do – but not my right side!

A DENTED IMAGE

Walking unsteadily can also attract unwelcome attention and potentially expose people to hurtful comments. As Roy recalled: 'I was walking down the street and there was a woman with a child saying "Come away from there. That man looks drunk to me!" which I felt was quite hurtful.' Perhaps it's not surprising that someone walking unsteadily is usually thought to be inebriated – the 'village drunk' as Pam described herself.

Driving

After a brain haemorrhage there is a legal requirement to inform the Driver and Vehicle Licensing Agency (DVLA) and it will only be possible to drive again with their approval. How long the driving licence is suspended for will depend on a number of factors – whether someone has developed epilepsy, for example, or if they had a fit at the time of the haemorrhage (Brain and Spine Foundation 2002). For someone who has been driving for years and perhaps using their car daily, this will be an important loss. Getting a driving licence for the first time can be an important marker of independence. Having it taken away can mean reverting to dependence on other people. For Janice, not being able to drive was 'ghastly'. Karen-Ann also hated the loss of independence:

> The driving was humungous for me; not having my car; having to rely on people . . . completely rely on people to get you back and forward to the doctor, to take you to your hospital appointment . . . I was so used to doing things on my own, being independent . . . planning them around friends and family so that they could take me, and making arrangements! That was really quite tough.

Sandra ended up being unable to drive for nearly two years as she had a fit just one month before she was due to get her licence back. Before that, driving had been one of her passions as epilepsy in childhood meant she was twenty before she had her first licence. However, she found a way of coping in a positive manner:

> I valued the fact that I was so capable without the car. It wasn't such a big deal any more and I was going to appreciate it that much more when I did get it back. At that stage [and] even

176

now, when I see someone limping or I see someone not well it just sort of snaps me into – I'm lucky!

Having the licence returned can be a significant marker on the journey of recovery, but getting back behind the wheel can be quite daunting. Wendy's licence was returned just under six months after her haemorrhage:

> But it was really scary . . . because suddenly even the very quiet roads seemed really busy and it's all the decisions about how fast are they going and can I pull out? And I think I must have been a very annoying driver to sit behind because I didn't want to go fast . . . I'd have to wait for everybody to pass from the opposite direction before I could pull out. I find driving, even now, very tiring; if I'm driving for more than about an hour, I feel my head going funny. I think it's the fact that you have to concentrate on so many things that you would normally do without realising!

Having a haemorrhage can affect someone's self-confidence in many ways including how confident they feel about driving again. As Shirley wrote: 'I do not yet have the confidence to drive too far; maybe I'm afraid I will get myself lost.' Perhaps this is also part of regaining the confidence to go outside the home because 'home' feels safer? Veronica found it helped her get back to driving if she had another driver with her in the car: 'Even in the early days when I got back to driving, I would like someone with me . . . I think this confidence thing takes a lot of working at.'

Leisure activities

Sports and exercise can be enjoyable and fulfilling and after a brain haemorrhage can play an important part in restoring not only physical health but also self-confidence and a sense of achievement. After an SAH it's a good idea for people to return to previous activities – as and when they feel able to. If someone is going swimming, initially they should take another adult along because of the risk of epilepsy. Contact sports that may involve blows to the head (e.g. rugby, boxing) are better avoided (Brain and Spine Foundation 2002; Foulkes 2004). A staged return to exercise is important. As Andrew found when he went swimming for the first time, too much too soon is not a good idea:

> Five to six weeks after, I wanted to get myself fitter because I was going back to work within 12 weeks . . . I did about four lengths and felt terrible – absolutely awful! That evening I felt dreadful; it was more than just exhaustion. I just felt ill. I did get a bit scared . . . but it didn't put me off and I left it for a few days and I went back very slowly; the next time wasn't quite so bad.

Sport can sometimes be incorporated into a physical rehabilitation programme, which as well as helping physical recovery can also engender a sense of achievement and be a social activity, if practised with other people. Graham was able to get back to golfing early on in his recovery from a stroke:

> I was still in rehab as an inpatient and the [physio]therapist said to me, 'Graham, you play golf,' and I said, 'I used to.' 'When your wife comes in next time, get her to bring in a golf club.' . . . and they took me up to the local golf club and said, 'What we want you to do now is just hit that golf ball.' . . . And it was marvellous; I was able to hit the ball, but where it went didn't matter. . . . I play very much one-handedly . . . It's been a life saver.

The Girl Guides movement had always been an important part of Karen-Ann's life. A year after her haemorrhage, she had to play a less active role than usual on the annual holiday with her Guides, but the following year, with encouragement, she completed an assault course involving crossing a rope bridge, wall climbing and abseiling – an achievement which left her 'absolutely delighted' and boosted her confidence that she would recover.

Although the haemorrhage can occur during a time of physical effort it can also happen when someone is going about their normal daily activities such as working, resting or sleeping. We do not yet know why it should happen on this particular day rather than on another (Brain and Spine Foundation 2002; Foulkes 2004). Despite this, if someone started to haemorrhage when they were exercising or playing sport they may find it difficult to resume the same activity because of associating it with what happened.

Although Veronica walked and swam in the first year, she only restarted going to the gym two years after her haemorrhage, and ended up enrolling in a different gym:

> I went back to the old gym but mentally, I couldn't; I didn't want to be there; that had bad memories for me, so I sort of wiped that one, pushed that one aside; I thought, well, I'm not going there. I just couldn't cope with that psychologically. I could probably have made myself, had I not had another choice available.

Seven months after the haemorrhage which started as he returned from running, although Brian has gone back to practising Tai Chi he doesn't feel able to resume an activity he'd enjoyed and which was a 'major part' of his life. For now: 'It's just a milestone that I will conquer; it's all about problem-solving; I am a problem solver by trade so this is a problem I can get around and fix it.'

Sometimes a previous leisure activity can be surprisingly helpful. Megan was able to recall her yoga teacher's advice which enabled her to relax during the diagnostic angiogram. Like many others, though, her head still feels vulnerable and a year later she says: 'I haven't gone back to yoga, but I think I must do that because I did enjoy it [but] I don't like the head hanging down bit.'

Spending more time at home is sometimes experienced as a positive factor during recovery. As Karen has found 'you're really safe in your own environment', but at the same time home-based activities can also give a focus and some structure to the day. Gardening is, as she says, 'very therapeutic':

> I've been enjoying the garden; it's been quite nice to rekindle things that I used to do years ago when the kids were small which I'd stopped doing . . . I give myself projects – like in the springtime, I was growing lots of vegetables from seed and it was something I could focus on and it just gives you a bit of purpose.

People sometimes used the time at home for activities which they felt would help their brain to recover, as well as being in an environment in which they felt comfortable. As Rosie explained:

> [Home] became a nest and I feel secure here; it's my place! . . .
> I'm quite happy to stay at home . . . I like sewing. I like doing
> craft things. I love doing puzzle books. This house gives me the
> opportunity to do jigsaws . . . now I'm quite happy to sit and do
> a jigsaw. I think I'm challenging my brain all the time.

Sometimes the haemorrhage can challenge people to find new activities. Patsy realises that there are many things she's had to give up but, as she says: 'You find an alternative . . . you find something that you *can* do.' Although she thinks doing word-search puzzles is 'a bit sad', she does find it helps to focus her mind.

Reading is a popular leisure activity for many people, but after the haemorrhage they can sometimes find it difficult to read as much or with the same enjoyment as before (Buchanan *et al.* 2000). Reading material may have to be more lightweight. This may be because of problems with vision or because it's difficult to concentrate. Reading for any length of time can be problematic. As Jan says, her concentration span isn't as good as it was before so now 'I might get through a chapter but that's enough.' For Jessica too, who was an avid reader and used to borrowing library books every few days: 'It's now two or three pages and I'm done. I haven't actually read a full book since my brain haemorrhage.'

Sometimes, when fatigue sets in later in the day, reading has to be fitted in earlier, so Patsy now finds she can concentrate on reading in the mornings, but further on in the day she simply can't continue. Although Graham can read, he's now unable to read blocks of text so has had to read line by line, which makes it almost impossible for him to read a book and follow the plot: 'So okay I've got that line and I've got that line but if I try to read it all, I wouldn't be able to do it – I'd forget what the dickens it's all about!' As recovery continues, people may find they are able to read more and perhaps move from magazines to books. As Karen-Ann explained, although she has to read at work, when she's at home: 'I haven't got that "sit down and read" back yet, but I've started reading a couple of trashy magazines and that's sparked up a bit of interest.'

Watching television – especially if it involves longer or more in-depth programmes – can also be affected. As Christine said, she tends to watch 'crap television' in the evenings as a way of relaxing and when she's too tired to do anything more demanding. People may watch shorter or simpler programmes and find they are unable to concentrate if there are any interruptions to their viewing (Buchanan *et al.* 2000). Rosie has found she has to watch television rather differently now:

> Things like *Silent Witness* on the telly; we record it and then I have to watch it again because I can't take all the things in all at the same time. I can't take it in at speed anymore, whereas I used to have no problem. I think your brain just wants a little bit, and then a rest and then a little bit and then a rest.
>
> (Rosie)

Megan still finds it hard to have a lot of noise around her. Although she used to have music playing or the radio on, she now quite likes it to be quiet: 'Unless there's anything I want to watch, I couldn't be bothered to turn it on; I wouldn't have it just for noise . . . for background or company.'

12

EMPLOYMENT

Changes and alternatives

Introduction

Employment can make a significant contribution to people's sense of well-being (C.R. Scott 2006). Having a job can enhance self-confidence and provide a valued role in today's society. Before their haemorrhage, most middle-aged or younger people will have been in full- or part-time paid employment so 'When can I go back to work?' is likely to be a very common question. At the time of the haemorrhage some people may have been in full-time work for many years, so the abrupt (even though often temporary) cessation of a key element in their day-to-day life can be difficult, as Karen-Ann found:

> Going back to work was a big goal . . . I was desperate to go back to work because that was part of being 'normal'. I'd always worked and not working was really quite hard. Not getting up in the morning and going to work! That's the only time I've ever had off work; I'd had a couple of days here and there and leave . . . So going back to work was it and I really liked my job. I really wanted to go back and do what I did.

Advice for patients and their families suggests that it's common 'to take quite a few months off work' (Brain and Spine Foundation 2005b: 16); 'at least three months, and often longer' (Foulkes 2004: 25). This doesn't stop people wanting to get back to work as this is often seen as a major stage of recovery.

Recent studies have found that on average people were able to return to work nine to 12 months after their haemorrhage (Hackett and Anderson 2000; Wermer *et al.* 2007) and three months was a minimum (C.R. Scott 2006). However, another earlier study found that people had gone back to work somewhat sooner than this:

> Most employed people had returned to work three months after their illness, initially part-time with most working full-time within weeks . . . Clearly for most people, returning to work at the earliest possible moment was one of the most therapeutic steps in their recovery. There was little benefit in protracting their convalescence beyond three months.
>
> (McKenna *et al.* 1989: 486)

As these researchers point out, returning to work can be very therapeutic, but with greater understanding of the more subtle effects of subarachnoid haemorrhage such as cognitive difficulties and mental fatigue, not everyone would share this view that a longer convalescent period can have 'little benefit'.

If people are able to return to work, when they are ready to do so will be an individual matter. It will depend on the nature of their job, how stressful or physically demanding it is, and whether or not they need to drive to get to the workplace. And, of course, it will depend on how their overall recovery progresses. The Brain and Spine Foundation (2002) makes the helpful suggestion that people need to use their common sense.

After a brain haemorrhage, if people do not return to their previous job, their future employment can change in one of several ways including: working fewer hours than previously (Buchanan *et al.* 2000; Wermer *et al.* 2007); moving to a lower level job with less responsibility (Buchanan *et al.* 2000; Cedzich and Roth 2005; Wermer *et al.* 2007); or moving to a completely different job (Morris 2001) which may or may not involve retraining.

When people retire after their haemorrhage, this may be a positive decision to adopt a different and perhaps more relaxed lifestyle. In other cases, returning to previous employment will simply not be possible due to the effects of the haemorrhage, so stopping work will be an enforced life change. When the haemorrhage occurred, some people may have already retired from work, or they may have been currently unemployed. In the latter case, some people will have decided not to seek work in the future, although many of them had not yet reached normal retirement age (Morris 2001). They will therefore be dependent on benefits or other financial support.

Studies of the employment-related outcomes have found considerable variations. This may be because the research was undertaken in different countries (e.g. UK, Netherlands, Australia, New Zealand, Canada, USA) with differing rehabilitation and support services and different cultural and social attitudes towards employment.

The next part of this chapter describes how people thought about and planned their return to work; how their employers responded to this; and people's experiences of their actual return to work. The chapter then looks at those people who did not return to their previous job – either as a positive choice or because this was not possible – and the kinds of alternative activities they took up (such as volunteering). It concludes with a brief discussion of the financial effects of unforeseen unemployment.

Planning a return to work

Contemplating a return to work can evoke mixed feelings. Being able to pick up the reins of a former job can feel like significant progress and achieving a major milestone in recovery, but it can also feel quite daunting. The benefits and challenges of this are described by Morris (2001) when he interviewed people approximately 16 months after their haemorrhage. Of those who had returned to work:

> The majority deemed themselves to be coping as well now as before the haemorrhage. Many of these patients reported feeling better once they had returned to work, even though several of them had found it harder than usual to start with and were often more fatigued than before, following a day at work.
>
> (Morris 2001: 8)

There are a number of possible reasons why survivors may want to return to work as soon as possible. They may be worried about whether their job will be held open, or they may want to prove to themselves that they are capable of doing their previous job and can only confirm this by being back at work. They may also find it difficult being at home and relatively inactive. Andrew was eager to return to his job in a local authority three months after his haemorrhage:

I felt vulnerable because other people had obviously managed without me being there and I thought, well they don't really

want me . . . obviously, I'm not needed! . . . I think I wanted to
prove I was still capable of doing what I'd done [before the
haemorrhage].

Unlike some others, no one was putting Andrew under any
pressure to return to work at three months. Indeed, most people
advised him to the contrary and suggested he waited until he had
recovered further:

I was being told by friends that 'You shouldn't go back now –
leave it another few months; wait until you're better' . . . [The
hospital] thought three months was the earliest and it was very
much up to me . . . I was foolish because I wanted to get back
to normal. And even then, I realise it was too soon . . . I should
probably have been off for another month or two.

Feeling anxious about returning to work is not uncommon. As
Roy realised, he needed to show his colleagues that the haemorrhage had not affected his ability to work, but he wasn't at all sure
he'd cope:

Part of the problem you have when you have an SAH is will I
be able to do what I did before? Can I cope? Will I be accepted
back? So there's a conflict between the two – you don't want to
go back but you need to go back; otherwise they'll think you
can't cope.

Cognitive impairments after a haemorrhage may be relatively
minor, but can still make contemplating a return to work a
worrying prospect. An important part of Brian's job with a major
IT company involved giving presentations where he needed to
present his ideas clearly, argue his case and convince his colleagues.
But as he explained:

I wasn't sure that I could have a discussion and put my point of
view across . . . you have to know what you're talking about
and if it's a good idea, then you have to put it across . . . people
aren't sceptics but they want to know if you've thought of all the
points of view for an argument so that was quite big! I thought

185

about the short-term memory problem. They said in hospital that I might have a short-term memory problem but it will get better, but for some reason I latched on to that.

Like Andrew and Roy, Brian was also concerned that having had a brain haemorrhage his employers might decide he was incapable of doing his previous job and it would be a case of 'No, don't let Brian do it! He's had an illness, give him a little corner and give him a cup of coffee and a doughnut and he'll be okay!' In the event, 20 seconds into his first presentation he was, he recalls, 'back in my comfort zone'.

In some cases, when they feel ready to work survivors will be looking for a new job but may be concerned that disclosing their recent medical history at an interview may compromise their chances of being offered employment. Feeling sufficiently confident to start applying for jobs may also be a potential barrier. After her haemorrhage, Kaz was very unsure whether she'd ever be able to work again, even though she was only in her late twenties: 'I just kept thinking, I bet I won't be able to go back to work.' When she started a part-time job eight months after the haemorrhage it was 'a big confidence booster', although she only told her prospective employer about the haemorrhage after she'd been offered the job.

Because timescales of recovery are so individual and depend on many different factors, it can be hard for someone to decide when they are going to return to work. When Christine asked at a hospital outpatient appointment when she should go back to work, she was told, 'When you are ready.' When she did return, three months after the haemorrhage, she realised it was probably too soon. Rosie received similar advice from her neurosurgeon – 'Don't go back to work until you feel ready' – but as she says 'How can you tell when you're ready? It's very difficult to know what that means.' Trying to decide when you've recovered sufficiently to return to work isn't easy, as Karen found when she tried going back to work at three months:

I must have been crazy, as I wasn't well enough physically or mentally. After two hours of hell, I left. What was I thinking of? Trying to work in front of a computer screen with double vision and telling everyone that I was fine . . . I went home in tears and it dawned on me that my recovery was going to be a lot longer than I thought.

Maybe if she'd been referred for an assessment by an employment rehabilitation service, her experience would have been less traumatic. As a recent survey of stroke survivors found, improved liaison between healthcare professionals and employers to negotiate a staged return to work could help more people get back to work (Different Strokes 2007).

Employers' involvement

After the haemorrhage, survivors can encounter very different reactions from their former workplace. Some people felt that they had been well supported by an employer who was sympathetic and understanding. Others, however, felt they had been put under pressure to return to work too soon and had sometimes been inadequately supported by their employers. Although Roy was entitled to six months off work on full pay, his manager wanted him to be back at work after four months. Roy feels this was too soon and would like to have been able to negotiate with his manager, particularly in terms of a phased return:

> My manager wanted to get me back to work . . . [he] wanted to get me back to work very very quickly, as in 'When are you coming back?' and he said 'Right, you can come back to work on the 17th of June . . . We'll have you back for half days and I will tell you what half days you're going to have. Every single day for half a day.'

Looking back, Roy is pleased he didn't opt for early retirement on medical grounds, but still feels that his employers were acting more in their own best interests:

> Getting back to work did me good because it made me move. It made me just go out there and strive to get back as best and quickly as I could. Looking back on it, if I'd been medically retired I would probably have just vegetated . . . it was probably the best thing to have happened to me but it was done in a very hard manner and I don't think it was for my benefit.

Although Andrew now recognises that returning to work after three months was probably too soon, his manager certainly didn't pressurise him: 'My boss came and saw me at home and obviously didn't push me to go back to work too soon – it was up to me.' Employers can also support someone's return to work by recognising that they may have possible difficulties which need to be addressed. Brian had been extremely concerned that the haemorrhage would affect his ability to work as before. He was worried that possible short-term memory problems would mean he needed to make notes during meetings. To facilitate this, they purchased him a hand-held computer. In the event he didn't need to use it but, as he says, their awareness of possible difficulties and willingness to help him were really important:

> I wanted a crutch and they were so supportive . . . 'We don't think you've got a problem, by the way, but we will go to this expense' . . . And for [his company] it's not that much, but if they gave one to everyone it would probably be quite a lot . . . I don't know whether they realise how good I feel about them making that small effort.

Having an employer who is sympathetic, supportive and prepared to adopt a flexible approach is extremely helpful, as in Tania's case. She knew during her recovery that she could eventually return, while she also recognised that her job would probably have changed:

> I always told them I was definitely interested in going back . . . and they left the space on the team . . . so I knew I had the place but as to what the job actually would be was unclear because things change when you're away . . . and now I've come back, I've not [got] exactly the same responsibilities and they have given me three months part-time just to acclimatise and that is the big thing about getting back to work.

It was also important, that they were able to arrange for her to have a phased return to work.

The return to work

A phased return to work

People like Tania can often manage a phased return to work – rather than either not working or having to go back to a full-time job – an 'either you're sick or you're well' approach. Fatigue is very common and may well increase when someone first goes back to work (Morris 2001), so starting back part-time, easing gradually back into the job, seems an obvious solution and one that worked well for Wendy:

> I needed to get back because I felt I had to try and do something normal, but it took me a long time to get into it properly. And then, after about five months, I started doing four days and I was on a four-day week for about 18 months; it took me quite a while to get back up to full-time . . . I was just having that extra day to sleep because the four days were making me so tired. I did find it very tiring [but] I was pleased in some ways because to me it was a big leap.

Karen-Ann was so eager to return to work that she kept telling her employer she'd be back – at first this month, then the next month, and then the month after that – but it wasn't until just over six months that her GP decided she was okay to return, although insisting this was not to be full-time:

> I did short hours. I went to work every day but for short periods of time. Then, after a month or so, I started to try and work longer hours and then I did some work at home if I couldn't get out of bed in the morning, which happens now as well . . . I can sit here and do a bit of work; they were really good to me. Sometimes I just actually can't get out of bed; I'm too tired.

This kind of gradual return can work really well, allowing people to build up their stamina and also giving their brain the opportunity to continue to heal and recover. Despite this, going back to work can still be stressful in the initial stages when, like Andrew, they may not feel confident but unable to say anything:

> When I did come back to work I was doing half-days . . . and then it's very easy for that to rapidly increase . . . People really didn't know how I felt that first week or that second week even, when I came back. I felt totally bewildered. I felt I was swamped.

189

I thought what the heck am I doing? I thought I couldn't really cope with it.

Timescales of recovery are very individual. Tania was unable to work for two years after her haemorrhage, but she and her employer have been able to negotiate a very gradual and gentle return to employment:

They've given me three months part-time just to acclimatise . . . I had HR [human resources] help me beforehand to arrange tentative meetings at work to get me back into the building and then it was another exercise to go and actually have a look at my desk on another day; it was all very emotional . . . it started off very lightly and the idea was to educate myself and read things and update myself and meet people.

Colleagues at work

Going back to work can be eased if colleagues are supportive, particularly in the early weeks. However, as Wendy discovered, other people may not appreciate the long-term nature of recovery, particularly if someone's difficulties are not immediately apparent:

They've been a lot more understanding at work; they've made a lot of allowances. Even now I think part of it is because [the haemorrhage] happened at work . . . and I think it was a case of they were just so pleased to see me, they would put up with anything. And they've been learning from it as well . . . But now I think it's pretty much a case of they know it happened but it's over with.

And as Andrew commented: 'Once people think you're back at work – hey, you're back in the job, at your desk, and that's it.' Perhaps it's difficult to get this right. If people are anxious to prove to themselves and others that they are still 'okay' and up to doing their job, they may be reluctant to say anything that indicates otherwise. Colleagues may unwittingly collude with this so everyone behaves as though things are back to normal. Maybe this is part of the 'get well soon' syndrome?

When Karen-Ann was returning to work, she heard from a colleague that her office were planning to have 'Welcome Back' balloons. This was the last thing she wanted. Despite the haemorrhage, she wanted to get back to normal:

> It will upset me too much because all I want to do is slide back in like I've never been gone. I didn't want to be the centre of attention. I didn't want it to be a fuss and a palaver.

Perhaps being the focus of attention could serve as too forcible a reminder of the 'palaver' when the brain haemorrhage happened – an abnormal event for most people and one they may prefer not to dwell on?

Survivors may sometimes be concerned that, rather than seeing them as 'back to normal' when they're back at work, their colleagues may think that the brain haemorrhage has damaged them in some way. At first John didn't want other people at his workplace to find out:

> Being open about what had happened was better than my initial feeling that I didn't want anyone to know. I winced slightly when I overheard a secretary at work say that I had been off work with 'a bleed on his brain' but it was no more than the truth. People could judge for themselves whether I was damaged goods, past the 'use-by' date.

Coping with cognitive problems and other difficulties

Cognitive difficulties such as short-term memory loss and problems with multitasking, together with ongoing fatigue, may still be issues when someone returns to work, but colleagues may not necessarily be aware that someone has these difficulties (Different Strokes 2007). Returning to a job that routinely requires someone to multitask can be problematic. Andrew realises, with hindsight, that he should have asked for more help from other people and let go of the reins:

> I was coming back to a sheer multitude of different things . . . whether it's getting work done at various locations on site to time and to budget, managing people, going to loads of

different meetings . . . it was a lot and I'd probably bitten off more than I could chew.

Christine had similar difficulties: 'I just couldn't do the multi-tasking that I could do [before the haemorrhage]. I couldn't do the juggling and people would be saying things and I'd just forget it.' Roy too had problems with walking and with short-term memory but when he went back to work he was determined to prove to his colleagues – and to himself – that he could still do his job, and do it well:

> It gave me the impetus to start saying – I'm back at work . . . It hasn't damaged me that much and I'm going to show them that I can do just as good a job as I did before . . . I do feel that after three or four months I was better than I was before because I made a conscious effort of being aware of everything that I was supposed to do; everything I was responsible for – apart from forgetting people's names!

When survivors are living with fluctuating levels of energy and having 'good' and 'bad' days, going back to work can be difficult if someone is unable to predict how they will be feeling the following week, or even the following day. Rosie, who had previously worked part-time, felt that because her fatigue and dizzy spells were not always predictable, she couldn't guarantee to her employer when she'd be able to work:

> I couldn't say 'I'll come in on Monday' because Monday I might not feel well and Tuesday might be better. So because I couldn't commit I was holding back. Even now, I don't think I would want to commit if I'd had a bad weekend, really bad fatigue, I couldn't have gone to work. If I'm unreliable then I'd be letting people down.

A change of role or a new job

Some people return to work and their job will be redefined or adjusted (Buchanan *et al.* 2000; Cedzich and Roth 2005; Wermer *et al.* 2007). This can be for an initial period. Six months after her haemorrhage, Megan returned to her nurse's job in a GP surgery, but didn't see many patients at first:

> I thought I'd go back and see how I felt about it . . . I was very much protected and could really choose what I was doing . . . They didn't book me sessions; I would go along and help with some of the admin work that had got left when I'd been away and I'd see the odd [patient] . . . and it was nice; I was practising in a very leisurely manner. [Now] I do two full days and a half day.

Tania also had a gradual return to work but 'now, only after three months are we at the stage of working out what my role is . . . it's nice to be given some small tasks to achieve'. However, as she points out, it can be difficult if 'confidence is seen as a bit of a minor fixable problem – "After you've been here a few weeks you'll be fine!"' Colleagues and managers may be unaware of how a brain haemorrhage can affect self-confidence.

Returning to work may not always go according to plan and sometimes people will decide to look for a new job when they realise things aren't working out as they'd hoped. Achieving this may take some time, as Lauren discovered. When her public sector employers suggested she return to work ten weeks after her haemorrhage, she agreed, but then, as she says, she 'crashed out of work' and had to take another month's sick leave. She returned to a different job in the same organisation where things worked out better and she felt her confidence was coming back. However, a move back to her original job didn't work out, so a year after her haemorrhage she moved to a completely new job. As she now realises, she should probably not have returned before six months, but 'hindsight is a wonderful thing, isn't it?'

These survivors were eventually able to return to work but this may not be the case for everyone. Some may decide to opt for retirement, while others will have no choice in the matter. Yet others may take up unpaid work, seeing it as a possible stage in returning to paid work eventually.

Alternatives to employment

Retirement

With people in their fifties being at the 'peak' age for brain haemorrhages, sometimes they may choose to retire rather than return to work. Janice had worked as a nurse for 30 years and at the time of her second haemorrhage was working part-time as a bank nurse in an accident and emergency department. Although she really loved her job, she decided not to go back because 'it was just a natural progression . . . a sort of hint that this was the time to stop; let's finish it now I thought, let's retire', and in the event she doesn't regret that decision.

For others, however, retirement is sudden and unplanned and any choice about whether or not to return to work isn't possible. After a serious haemorrhagic stroke, Graham still hoped that he would recover sufficiently to return to his previous demanding job in a design and manufacturing consultancy. Having been advised that he'd be doing well if he got back within 50–75 per cent of how he was before the stroke, he then realised that his goal of returning to work would not be possible:

> I was neither physically able nor mentally able to do it because the work I did was highly demanding and required hours of concentration. And that's been really the biggest thing that I have not come to terms with, having to pack up work, because you lose that feeling of usefulness and purpose, because you need a purpose to get up in the morning.

Despite this sudden and major loss, however, Graham has developed a new and different lifestyle. As well as resuming his golfing, he has become a trustee of the Val Hennessy Trust (see Appendix B) and visits a rehabilitation centre regularly where he befriends and supports stroke patients.

Finding alternatives to paid employment

Resuming previous employment may not be possible for a number of different reasons: the return to work may have been premature; physical and/or cognitive difficulties may make this impossible; an employer may decide the person can't return; or someone may decide to make a career change for positive reasons.

Seven months into recovery, David was still unsure whether he'd be able to resume his previous career as a successful chef. He'd tried to go back to work, but when things didn't work out he lost his job, although he feels he would probably have needed a year to get back up to speed. Faced with what he describes 'an enforced career change', he's decided to use his time out of employment to possibly retrain for a new career. Whatever kind of work he chooses to do in the future, he's determined that things will work out – 'I'm going to win whatever way' (and David did manage to complete the London Marathon six months after his haemorrhage).

Physical and/or cognitive difficulties can make it difficult or impossible for someone to return to their previous job. Before her haemorrhagic stroke Pam was working as a nurse, but realised she would be unable to continue because of her physical difficulties and concern that she might make errors with handing out patients' medication. She had, however, already started training as a psychotherapist and despite the effects of her stroke and with considerable determination, she has been able to continue her training and is working with clients.

Voluntary work can be a useful stepping stone to paid employment, enabling people to build up their self-confidence and test out their skills and abilities. It also provides a sense of purpose and structure in day-to-day life. Christine returned to work four months after her haemorrhage but found she was struggling. Working two days a week, she was inevitably doing more hours and fatigue was a major problem. When the company's reorganisation meant she was made redundant, this came as a relief and she started working at her local infants school on a voluntary basis:

Possibly the worst environment for head injury! But that was really good therapy for me in actual fact. Because I was in the reception class it was simple . . . lots of glueing and sticking and painting and glueing and it was lovely! The girl I worked with was fantastic for my self-esteem. 'Oh, you're just perfect at this!' and she would be constantly bolstering my ego.

After volunteering Christine then got a job working on the infants' literacy project and subsequently moved to a full-time job in the senior school. Five days a week proved too much but she now works Mondays to Wednesdays: 'I recover Thursday, Friday and I'm good at the weekend for the family . . . From my point of view it works – sort of giving something and getting something back, to watch them achieve . . . I find that very satisfying.' Through volunteering Christine has changed career, but she can still work part-time and contribute to family life.

The type of work someone was doing when they had a brain haemorrhage sometimes means it will be impossible for them to take up where they left off. Eight years ago Vernon was working 'round the clock' as a builder until he suddenly collapsed at work. For the first three or four years he spent time with Headway where, having started out as a service user he became a volunteer and then worked as a part-time assistant manager. He has subsequently trained and worked as a counsellor, and is currently training to work with young offenders.

Prior to his haemorrhage, Scott and a colleague had set up their own company and had just won a large contract. Despite attempting to do some company work when he first came out of hospital, he's had to let go of something in which, he says, 'we not only had a lot invested financially but emotionally as well . . . but I've closed the door on that'. Although he's not yet been able to return to paid employment, Scott has been more involved in his sons' education and spending time at their school. He is wondering whether he might eventually train to become a teacher.

When a return to work in the near future isn't possible, there is at least time and space to think about possible alternative futures. Patsy realises that fatigue and difficulties with concentration meant she would be unable to go back to her previous job in banking, but feels that what has happened could present her with new opportunities:

> I always felt I wanted to do something which was more useful, even then. So perhaps I had the brain haemorrhage for a reason? I know when I worked at the bank, I used to think to myself I'd really like to work in a hospital or . . . Perhaps this was all meant to be? . . . perhaps out of the haemorrhage something else is happening to my life.

Patsy now volunteers at a day centre for people with a range of disabilities, but she has also been on the NHS's Expert Patients course (which helps people self-manage chronic or long-term health conditions) and one thing led to another:

> I did the six weeks and they came to me at the end and said 'We think you'd make a brilliant tutor!' That was hard work – the person that can't read, taking in information, doing things – I passed it! . . . You know I was saying to you [in the interview] 'I exist' but I try to make the most of what I've got . . . there's

lots of things I'd like to do now that I can't do so you have to accept that and try and do the things you can.

Patsy still hopes she may get a job again one day, possibly through her voluntary work, but has been able to use her experiences of illness and recovery to explore new avenues.

The financial effects of unemployment

Although the interviews did not include any questions specifically about people's financial status, several people did mention this, usually in the context of talking about employment – either their own or that of the main family carer. Mezue and colleagues have suggested that because of the psychosocial disruption which follows brain haemorrhage 'there would be considerable economic costs to the families' (Mezue *et al.* 2004: 137). Even when people are on full pay, perhaps for six months after they had had to stop work, this may not be long enough if they have not yet recovered sufficiently to return to work. They may be still grappling with cognitive, physical and emotional issues when their pay is reduced; benefits (which are unlikely to match someone's previous salary) may be the only alternative source of income.

When someone has been able to resume work, their salary may be lower than before. In Christine's case, she found it difficult at first to accept that her husband would now be the main provider:

My full-time pay ran out quite quickly so I was then on incapacity benefit very very quickly . . . I've been able to slow down on the work front so the income I bring in now as a teaching assistant is peanuts and so the pressure is very much on Mike to be the main provider. So that made me feel guilty . . . but we've always talked everything through so he doesn't feel that . . . it's pressure I put on myself really.

When sickness pay is coming to an end, the survivor may feel they need to return to work. Wendy feels that she returned to work too soon, but as she says: 'I went back because I was on full-time sick pay for six months and I wanted to go back before I started losing pay.' Even when someone has not been the main breadwinner in the family, but has contributed financially, the unexpected loss of employment can affect previous patterns of expenditure. As Karen explained: 'You've been used to having a certain standard of living and . . . you're used to having x amount of money and being able to spend that.' Although she has not yet returned to work, she says 'financially, probably that would be the only reason at the moment that I would go back [to work]'.

When a partner or spouse becomes the survivor's main carer, if they were already in employment they may well need to take a substantial amount of time off work (Pritchard *et al.* 2004). If their caring role extends beyond a few months, they may also have to change jobs to accommodate this, affecting the family income. Pam's husband left the police service in order to look after her and moved to a job with less pay and responsibility and they no longer had Pam's income from nursing.

A sudden and unplanned reduction in the family's income can have a significant impact, particularly when the survivor had previously made a significant contribution to the overall income. Heather, who had held down a well-paid job before her haemorrhage, now finds that 'money has been a massive problem for us recently'. Whereas she, her husband and their young son could afford to go out regularly, now, she says: 'We don't have any money and we don't really do a great deal; not like we used to be able to.'

Claiming benefits can be lengthy and time-consuming and, as Scott found, it was some time before the Benefits Agency accepted that his wife would be speaking on his behalf as, at first, he was unable to use the phone himself. Having previously run his own business, 'now that the benefits are in place we're actually more secure financially, even though there's less money coming in [and it's] more regular'.

Part IV

MAKING SENSE
OF IT ALL

13

FINDING WAYS THROUGH RECOVERY: WHAT HELPED

Introduction

This chapter is about 'finding ways' because there isn't 'a way' – a one size fits all – to recover. As I explained in Chapter 1, this book is not intended to be a manual for recovery or a comprehensive guide, but towards the end of each interview I asked people to talk about what they felt had helped them to recover. This chapter draws together their responses and for those who have recently had a brain haemorrhage perhaps they will find ideas here which resonate for them. For those providing care and support services, the ideas set out may also offer some useful ideas about how these services can better meet people's needs.

Survivors talked about how they had looked for ways of recovering that would work for them. As Andrew said: 'Different people will look in different directions.' Lauren decided that approaching her recovery from a cognitive perspective worked for her 'like dealing with things that are in front of you that are hurdles . . . I sat and did it on my own because I didn't turn to other people to tell me how to run my life.' Vernon's starting point was to adopt a 'positive outlook, then to become motivated to find your own ideas and what works for oneself'.

Survivors have also described elsewhere what has helped them to recover, including, family and friends (Chapter 10), meeting other survivors (Chapter 6), rehabilitation services (Chapter 6), managing cognitive difficulties (Chapter 8) and emotional difficulties (Chapter 9). Before describing survivors' experiences, I briefly discuss some theoretical frameworks that seem to underpin those experiences – coping strategies, locus of control and resilience.

Thinking about recovery: some theoretical frameworks

Coping strategies

The use of coping strategies can play a part in helping people recover from illness or injury and may make a positive contribution to the rehabilitation of those who have sustained a traumatic brain injury or who are recovering from other neurological conditions (Moore and Stambrook 1992). From the interviews, it was clear that people had used a range of coping strategies to help themselves recover, including problem-solving and emotional strategies which Taylor (1998) describes as follows:

> the specific efforts, both behavioural and psychological, that people employ to master, tolerate, reduce or minimise stressful events. Two general coping strategies have been distinguished: *problem-solving* strategies are efforts to do something active to alleviate stressful circumstances, whereas *emotion-focused* coping strategies involve efforts to regulate the emotional consequences of stressful or potentially stressful events.
>
> (Taylor 1998, emphasis added)

Problem-solving strategies would include focusing on doing something about the situation, taking action to try and make the situation better, getting help and advice from other people, and getting comfort and understanding from another. Emotion-focused strategies, on the other hand, would include accepting the reality of what has happened, looking for something good in what is happening and trying to make what has happened seem more positive (Carver 1997).

The ways in which people cope with their recovery will depend to some extent on their personal style (e.g. some cope more actively than others), the nature of the event, and the degree of control which they have over physical health problems, which may feel less controllable (Taylor 1998). Carleen Scott's (2006) study of survivors of subarachnoid haemorrhage found that their use of coping skills could have a positive or negative impact on their quality of life, in terms of their general outlook, emotional well-being, cognitive functioning, relationships, leisure and social participation, and work. These she concluded 'require focus for rehabilitation in order to increase the patients' quality of life [and] it is also imperative that patients are given the tools in order to cope with their change in quality of life' (2006: 44). Neurological centres and rehabilitation services could work with survivors by helping them acquire positive coping skills to aid their recovery.

Locus of control

The concept of locus of control suggests that we may come to believe that what happens to us is the direct result of our own actions ('internal locus of control'), due to the actions of others, or determined by fate, luck or chance ('external locus of control'). Issues of control were explored in Chapter 9 (pp. 147–8) which described the difficulties people sometimes experienced after their haemorrhage: the realisation that they'd had no control over its occurrence and that they had (temporarily at least) been forced to relinquish control over some key areas of their life (e.g. driving, working) where they'd been accustomed to being in control. In these circumstances, people were having to come to terms with the fact that the haemorrhage and its immediate effects were not within their control. Accepting what had happened could therefore be a healthy and less stressful coping strategy (see below).

When it came to dealing with their recovery some survivors were able to draw on their belief in an internal locus of control so how they recovered would be largely in their hands. This is not to reject the help and support of other people, but rather describes a general approach which some survivors used.

Resilience

The concept of resilience relates to both coping strategies and locus of control but is also relevant here. Being resilient is about being able to do well despite facing difficult conditions in life, adapting to misfortunes and setbacks without resorting to negative or unhealthy coping strategies such as alcohol or substance abuse, or denying that a setback has occurred. Although Vanistendael (1996), who developed and elaborated this concept, focused initially on the needs and rights of children, his ideas have had increasing currency in other areas and with people of all ages.

Fostering resilience relates to five areas of people's lives: their social support networks; the capacity to discover meaning in life; the feeling of having control in life; having self-esteem or positive ideas about oneself; and a sense of humour which can integrate the suffering. It is clear from this that resilience can help us better understand how people may recover from subarachnoid haemorrhage.

Resilience involves harnessing our inner strengths, adapting to stress and change and reaching out to others. It is not about ignoring feelings of sadness and loss, always having to be strong, or being distant, cold and unfeeling (Mayo Clinic 2005). The good news is that we can teach ourselves to become more resilient. As Patsy said: 'Perhaps I had an easy life before and something like this just pulls you up . . . I think I'm a stronger person than I thought I was.' Having outlined some theories which seem to relate to survivors' experiences, the remainder of this chapter describes this mainly in their own words.

Approaches to recovery

There were several different strands to the ways in which survivors approached their recovery, characterised by these mental attitudes: a determination that they would recover; wanting to turn something negative into a positive; taking control over their recovery; and finding reasons to recover. These attitudes echo those of a group of survivors interviewed several years after their haemorrhage where 'the overriding impression gained . . . was how well many seemed to have recovered and how positive they were about their lives' (Ogden *et al*. 1997: 31). Perhaps, the researchers speculated, this was because they had survived a condition where the death rate is 50 per cent and had then coped with major neurosurgery.

The word 'determination' cropped up frequently in the interviews. Despite the effects of their haemorrhage, there was a strong resolve to recover. Jan, who describes herself as being 'strong willed', feels this helped her recover because, as she says:

> I was so determined that I was going to get back to normal and I'd be well . . . I suppose I could have just thought that's the end of my life but it isn't, you know? I think you tend to think you've got to do more now, you've got to prove things because you were on death's door and you're not now.

Graham, like Jan, also had to spend months in a residential rehabilitation centre before he was able to return home. For

Graham it was a matter of working on his recovery to meet the goals he'd set himself:

> Just never give up; never give up at all . . . if you're just going to sit there and sulk about it, you'll be there for ever and I didn't want that. I wanted to get back on the golf course and I wanted to get out and do other things and I wanted to drive.

Pam feels that she has become 'a lot more positive [and] a lot more determined' since her haemorrhagic stroke and this has affected the way she has focused on her psychotherapy training where, despite some continuing difficulties, she is now determined to do well – and to prove to herself that her stroke has not affected her academic ability:

> I think I could be easily sidetracked before and I could very easily be sloppy; I could do sloppy work with my studying because it was sort of, well, it doesn't matter . . . it bloody well matters now! I'm more determined to do well academically . . . so there must be a fear there that perhaps something happened intellectually because I do have to try harder now.

Determination was often accompanied by a recognition that if they were to recover well, this would be mean hard work. As Patsy reflected: 'They [the neurosurgeons] do the op, but you do the hard work . . . It doesn't just happen; it's because we make it happen; we work hard . . . everything is hard work now.' It also meant that the survivor was taking charge – exercising control over their recovery. As Roy explained:

> I don't want to just sit back in a chair and say 'I've had a brain haemorrhage – everybody help me' because I don't want to do that . . . 'Oh you're so lucky to have survived!' okay, that might be the case, but it's not just luck any more; now it's down to me to sort it out.

A year after her haemorrhage, Patsy was very involved in planning her daughter's wedding. Jan found her grandchildren were her reason for recovering: 'My main goal was to be there for my grandchildren and especially the baby that had just been born; I wanted to see her grow up . . . so that has stimulated me to get better.' Lesley had been accepted on a psychotherapy training course before the haemorrhage:

> Yes, it provided me with something to fight for, because I was very aware that I was going to have to fight with my brain to get it going again . . . I'm a very determined person so I was determined that I would recover; I saw no reason why I shouldn't.

Even a relatively modest goal can make a positive difference. When a friend said to Rosie that she'd never be able to make her usual Christmas visit to Cornwall two months after her haemorrhage, she was determined to prove him wrong, but this also gave her a reason to recover:

> I thought, right, I will then! And I think that got me through it; the determination of the things I had to do, the things I had to look to, actually started to make me forget about what had happened . . . it gave me a goal.

The coping strategy of 'positive reframing' was also important for some survivors – trying to see what had happened to them in a different light, to make it seem more positive and looking for something good in what was happening (Carver 1997). For Brian, having a positive mental attitude was critical and writing about his experiences on the internet he called it The Positive Blog:

> because I try and put a positive view on everything . . . a lot of people came back and said 'You're' right!' If you look at it, there's a positive view about everything . . . and I look at my recovery and the positive things about recovery and what I can do . . . mental attitude is the thing that helps you recover, isn't it?

Rosie too, was determined to find something positive: 'I'm not one to put it behind me and forget that it's happened. I'm going to make the best out of my experience!' And for Graham, using his experiences in a positive way, was his way of coping:

That's how I coped with it. What can I do with what's happened to get something out of it? . . . It's a negative thing that happens, can we turn that around into a positive? And that's what I did. That's what I still do.

Having included people's experiences of how their positive attitudes helped their recovery, Lesley, while agreeing that it worked for her, also sounds a note of caution: 'My positive attitude was hugely helpful . . . [but] I think for someone who has a tendency to see the negative, it would be a horrendous experience.' As other chapters make clear, there are many difficulties along the way.

Setting goals and marking achievements

The survivors were frequently using planning and active coping strategies which would enable them to recover, and putting these strategies into action (Carver 1997). They described how important they had found it to set themselves goals. This seemed to work not only by helping them to recover physically and psychologically, but also meant they had taken control of their recovery which in turn helped to increase their self-confidence and self-esteem. As Rosie explained:

You have to have goals and aims and you have to decide what it is that you want to do, what you want your future to be and then construct it . . . structuring them gradually . . . it's goals and aims that get you through it.

As Robert McCrum wrote: 'Throughout my recovery, I found it helpful to set myself limited short-term personal goals of the kind I had a reasonable expectation of achieving' (1998: 141). Describing their goal-setting activities, survivors emphasised the importance of realistic and achievable objectives. They were, in fact, using the SMART acronym: specific, measurable, attainable, realistic and timely.

Whatever you do, set yourself a target that you think is realistic, something that you can measure as well and it's achievable . . . but don't be worried if you have to re-set your targets. You have to push the boundaries a little bit each time but if you don't feel up to it, then don't overdo it . . . the problem came for me when I was overdoing things physically. It's trying to set a realistic goal, I think.

(Andrew)

Setting realistic targets, rather than setting yourself up to possibly 'fail', was important:

Don't set yourself ridiculous targets! I remember saying in hospital at the time that I will never, ever, shout at my children again, but that lasted – five minutes?

(Christine)

Graham was advised:

Don't set your target too high! And I found that was good advice because all the way through, I find if you set yourself goals that you can achieve that sense of achievement is so much greater than setting yourself a goal that you can't achieve because then if you don't get it, you get the disappointment.

(Graham)

Even modest goals, which Lesley described as 'bite-sized chunks', could make a big difference and helped people to pace their recovery:

It would even be the stupid little things like say, today I'm going to walk to the house three doors away. And I'd do it and then it would be four doors away or I'd go to the postbox or something . . . And it was even things like, this morning I'm going to put my own socks on, rather than have my husband do it.

(Patsy)

By planning specific and realistic goals, and attaining what they'd set out to do, the result is often a great sense of achievement. Lauren described how right from the start she was giving herself 'marks' as she met the targets of her daily programme of going out, going for a swim, and so on. Karen-Ann tried to do 'everything' for the first three months, but having set more realistic goals she was then able to celebrate an achievement, though she was aware this might not seem a big deal to other people:

> I changed the continental quilt; I got the quilt inside the quilt cover and pillows inside the pillowcases – it took me three hours! But when I finished – the sense of satisfaction, you'd swear I'd just got a Master's degree in bed making! I was absolutely over the moon that I'd done that all by myself . . . it sounds so trivial, doesn't it? Most people would take for granted making a bed but that was quite a milestone for me . . . once I'd done those buttons up at the bottom of the quilt, I cried! But cried with a big smile on my face . . . I've done it. Brilliant!

Like Karen-Ann, Christine found – or refound – happiness in what to others may seem an unremarkable achievement. Refinding happiness was a turning point after a difficult time. She recalls a day out with her husband:

> I can remember laughing. We went down to [the coast] for the day and I remember thinking, gosh, I hadn't realised how much I used to laugh. And I played on one of those things on the piers – one of those grab things – and I actually grabbed, I think it was the pink cat Bagpuss . . . and it was almost like a turning point – it was a beautiful day and it was just the two of us and we walked and walked all around by the sea – it was a positiveness that sort of developed from then on – I can win something!

Acceptance and adjustment

This important and positive coping strategy involves accepting the reality of what has happened and being able to live with the outcomes (Carver 1997). Of course people know – often soon after the event – that they have had a brain haemorrhage, but accepting what has happened and finding ways of living with the consequences can be rather different. Denial in the very early days can be helpful and protective, but if it persists over time, it can be difficult for survivors to accept what they have been through and move on. As the reality of what has happened begins to set in, it can still take time for people to accept that the haemorrhage had happened and that their life will probably have changed – sometimes permanently. As Patsy said:

> I think it takes a long while – acceptance. It took me a long time to accept what has happened. I did the Expert Patients course and I started to think, okay, well this has happened to me but you've still got something to give. My life will never be the same, I don't think, but I've got a new life, a different life! I know in my heart I'm never going to be the person I was pre-haemorrhage but I'm this new person now . . . I just can't do everything the same.

Whatever 'good' or positive may have come out of the haemorrhage – and that is the subject of the next and final chapter – this may perhaps help people to accept what has happened. For Karen-Ann, there was a lot of questioning first:

> Acceptance that it's happened; that took a while. Why did it happen to me? . . . all of that went through my mind for a bit . . . Once you've accepted it's happened and that things aren't going to be the same as what they were before, nothing's so bad. I can't say I'm glad it's happened, but it has changed my perspective on some things. [But] I would have preferred not to have had my perspective changed by something quite as calamitous as that!

Acceptance includes being able to live with any resulting difficulties. As Shirley wrote: 'I'm able to cope with my shortcomings and, most importantly, I am happy.' Setting achievable goals helped people with their recovery, but with some difficulties it may be a question of acknowledging them and finding ways of adjusting to them. As Christine found, with continuing mental fatigue and cognitive difficulties, she could organise her life to accommodate them:

> It's the adjusting to everything I suppose. Now I've recognised that – which took a while – then if I stop and 'give in' to [fatigue], I can recover quickly. The only way to improve – it's my acceptance.

Trevor Powell suggests that being able to accept and adjust to changes is an important marker of progress:

Although everybody is different, there seem to be a number of possible signs of long-term emotional adjustment when the person does feel more at ease with themselves and their situation. They might be able to identify and list their main problems that are the result of the brain injury, showing some insight and understanding . . . A further sign of progress is that of growing acceptance and a lowering of their expectations on themselves. This results in the person being able to say, 'Realistically I can't do that as I used to. I can't do it that way. I have to do it differently.' This does not mean stopping doing things but means doing them differently. This also means forgiving oneself when mistakes are made.

(Powell 2004: 199)

Doing things differently – adapting to changed circumstances – helped Patsy adjust to the fact that since the haemorrhage she has been unable to look upwards. Despite this, she still managed to see the famous Michelangelo ceiling in the Sistine Chapel by walking round with a mirror and, perhaps more importantly, using a special mirror, she is able to drive again. As she says: 'You do find ways if you really want to.' Similarly, Karen has had to adjust to problems (in her case with eyesight), and 'do things in a different way'. They are like the survivors in Ogden *et al.*'s (1997) study who displayed 'a willingness to adapt to their problems and get on with life' (1997: 31).

Writing about newly acquired disability, Larner makes the useful point that people can find it more helpful if they learn to 'manage' rather than 'master' aspects of their disability (Larner 2005: 37). Survivors can therefore accept any changes but also feel that they can find ways of adjusting to them. Janice makes the point that acceptance also means being kind to yourself: 'You've got to realise that this thing has happened and things have changed and you've got to adjust and change your life and make allowances for yourself, so be good to yourself.' Treating yourself with compassion is important.

Self-compassion

Survivors struggling with low self-esteem can find it difficult to treat themselves compassionately and to follow Janice's advice to be good to themselves. Self-esteem is often seen as being dependent on what we achieve – do something well and your self-esteem will soar – but only seeing it as related to achievement may be questionable: 'Developing self-esteem can imply developing beliefs about abilities to achieve goals. Although this can be laudable and valuable, it may not address the issue of acceptance for failures' (Gilbert and Irons 2005: 292). Developing a compassionate mentality towards the self would include: 'sympathy and empathy for one's own life situation and experiences; the ability to feel "warmth" for the self; the ability to adopt a forgiving attitude to the self' (p. 292). Janice also talked about 'making allowances' for oneself. Vernon found that meditation had helped him to be 'non-judgemental' towards himself. To put this yet another way, as Pam suggested, thinking about her own experiences:

> I think what might be helpful to other people is – if you get it wrong, it's okay . . . I have had empathy for myself but not that wallowing in self-pity . . . it's really self-compassion isn't it . . . it's about being kind to yourself and being gentle with yourself.

Having already described how survivors had marked their achievements, it may sound rather paradoxical to start talking about allowing oneself to get things wrong and to be forgiving of one's failures. After Lesley had talked about how she was determined 'to kick [her brain] back into shape' she recognised the seeming contradiction because 'in some ways I'm more compassionate with myself which goes exactly against what I've just been saying'. Perhaps recognising this may be helpful for survivors?

Recent studies have drawn attention to the importance of treating oneself kindly and with compassion when faced with difficult life events. The researchers found that self-compassion can help to lessen the anger, depression and pain that can result from adversity and can allow people to accept what has happened (Leary *et al.* 2007). Being compassionate towards oneself can include caring for your body as well as your mind.

'Listen to your body'

If there's one piece of advice many survivors remembered being given, it was: 'Listen to your body' (with possible subtext 'so when you're tired, take a rest'). Monitoring their physical state seemed to be a barometer of how much – or how little – people should attempt to do, particularly in the early stages of recovery. Physical and mental fatigue are 'your body's way of telling you to slow down' (Brain and Spine Foundation 2005b: 5). This sounds pretty straightforward, but before their haemorrhage people may have taken it for granted that their body would generally behave, that it usually wouldn't let them down. Following this advice was easier said than done and although many survivors wanted to pass it on, they'd often only learned the importance of listening to their body by finding out what happened when they hadn't followed their own advice. Being able to give yourself permission to 'listen to your body' and rest when necessary is not always easy. As Wendy suggested:

> You do need to get the balance right . . . It's hard to do if you're stubborn, then you want to keep going. It's almost like you've got to prove that you're okay and you've got to keep going. [If] anybody else was doing it, I'd say to them 'Stop! Sit down and have a rest, take it easy, take the day off. You don't have to do this.' But because it's you, you can't, you've got to keep going. On my good days I do give myself permission and I do think, yes, you've been through a rough time. But then on my not good days I don't do that.

Janice was another survivor who found this difficult because she wanted things to get back to normal as quickly as possible:

> You think, I must be better now. I must get on now and do this and start that . . .and, I think you need to listen to your body and say, no, I must sit down now and take it easy and not push myself too much because I was impatient to be back to my old self.

Megan, on the other hand, really enjoyed the novelty of going to bed during the day and feels this really helped her to recover:

> I used to love my afternoon nap. This started at the [hospital] and when I came home I thought I'd continue that, and whatever happened, I used to say to people if they'd ask to come and see me 'Not between one and two o'clock' and I

think it did help, just going to bed and resting. I've never been a person to sleep in the day at all, so that was nice.

Tania, like many others, found that while rest was important it was balanced alongside a need to actively work at her recovery:

You've got all this spare time and not much energy to do anything with it . . . I had an old-fashioned Jane Austen type convalescence, sitting in the garden, just seeing friends for tea – just having visitors or just keeping to your routine and taking some rest. And knowing that if you're tired, you take half an hour or an hour, sit down, then you do feel a bit better eventually and not keep ploughing on. But you can't stop yourself keeping active and testing your limits so you recover.

Taking relaxation breaks somewhere quiet for 20 to 30 minutes several times a day can be helpful (Brain and Spine Foundation 2005b), but again this is something people may have never tried before. Vernon started using relaxation tapes and CDs which he found helpful:

Sometimes wanting to sit down and block off and not have to concentrate on anything and just relax the brain . . . whereas I would never relax before my brain haemorrhage . . . it was something I had to do for myself, to relax.

If rest, rest and more rest was the mantra of recovery, some survivors also mentioned that working on their physical fitness had helped them to recover. David, who ran the London Marathon less than a year after his haemorrhage, believes that 'being fit and staying fit' has been central to his recovery. Others mentioned that their physical recovery was helped by increasing activities such as swimming – and being unable to drive for some months could mean discovering the pleasure of walking.

Since his haemorrhage, John has been 'absolutely compliant' with his blood pressure lowering medication because, he says: 'I am determined that, although I will be carried off eventually by something, it will not be by a blown gasket if I can help it!' Restrictions following brain haemorrhage can be irksome but can also contribute to physical well-being. Drinking at pre-haemorrhage levels can result in survivors having headaches or feeling sleepy or drunk more quickly (Foulkes 2004). Although not everyone had accepted this advice, some people had reduced their alcohol consumption during recovery and had continued to drink less.

Humour

Strange as it may sound, using humour by joking and making fun of the situation can be a positive coping strategy (Carver 1997). This is borne out by Ogden and her colleagues where jokes and humorous comments during their interviews with survivors 'were suggestive of a positive attitude to recovery' (Ogden *et al.* 1997: 31). Boss suggests that 'humor is an acknowledgement of things being the crazy way that they are. If we remain humorless, we are without hope. If we can begin to laugh, we have the capacity to find hope' (2006: 189). Humour can foster resilience.

The interviews for this book had their moments of humour when we could laugh together. Janice called her brain haemorrhage 'my stroke of luck' and Scott talked about having 'a little stir to my brain'. Because the effects of a brain haemorrhage aren't always visible, someone suggested that it would help to wear a badge saying 'I've had a brain haemorrhage'. And Graham, who described the physiotherapists at the rehab centre as 'physio-terrorists', reckoned that 'what's really got me through it all is humour'. Using humour, by cracking jokes, for example, can help people survive in a traumatic and otherwise anxiety-provoking situation which could become too overwhelming. This helped Tania to cope after she left hospital, but perhaps this also stemmed from a sense of relief, having survived a life-threatening event:

> I think my reaction was a little bit like a survival instinct, to become like a comedian! I was just cracking jokes all the time. I think I've heard it referred to [as] a kind of post-op hysteria thing, that everything seemed to be funny and quipping puns all the time. I just needed to laugh, I think that was it – just to cope with the shock.

Experiences in a neurosurgery unit can also sometimes be laughed about afterwards. David's haemorrhage started on a trip abroad, and although his wife had told him about the brain surgery, staff hadn't been able to explain what an angiogram involved:

The next thing I know, this nurse comes up and starts shaving my groin, and I'm going . . . there's a four feet difference here between the two places! I'm going 'no no' and they were going 'it's okay, it's okay'.

When David came back from theatre, there was a further misunderstanding:

The first thing I see when I open my eyes is this Benedictine monk at the end of the bed . . . he's got the Bible in his hand and he's throwing water over me. I just thought 'I'm dead, I'm dead – I've popped it!' and I remember opening my eyes and going 'I'm not dead! I'm not dead!' . . . such a vivid memory.

Humour during recovery can involve striking a balance. As Rosie explained:

You've got to draw the line between making light of it and actually mocking it, because you don't want to make people think that you're trivialising it, because it's not a trivial thing, but it's the way I get through because if I don't laugh, I'll cry. I think you've got to have a certain amount of humour to get you through. You need positive things to overcome the negative because there's so much negative and if you dwell on it and take it too seriously it's going to inhibit your recovery, I'm sure . . . It's definitely my way of coping.

Vanistendael (1996) suggested that a sense or humour can foster resilience when someone can recognise their problems, treat themselves with tenderness and accept their failures. Survivors sometimes joked about their cognitive or physical difficulties, rather than being self-critical, but it could also be a way of explaining to others why you don't always get things right. As Patsy said: 'I take the Mickey out of myself a bit more. I think you have to! I'll call myself all these silly names and I just say to people "You know! Brain's not working properly!" or something and we just laugh.'

Joking can also be a gentle or light-hearted way of explaining to other people what has happened and even turning it to your advantage. As Brian explained:

I think I'm having fun with it! . . . I'm having fun saying 'Oh, I can't do that because of brain surgery!' . . . Maybe I'm going to be the first brain surgery comedian – I don't know. [It's] playfulness, yes. . . . I've got an excuse. If something goes wrong, you just lift your hairline and go 'Look! Look at the scar!' I used that a lot going shopping! 'I'm not going to carry this – look at the scar!' . . . The number of times you say, 'I'm recovering from brain surgery' and they don't believe you and you just show the scar and they go 'Oh, really!' And they treat you really well.

Joking with people who don't know about the brain haemorrhage can, however, be a bit risky as Wendy found:

I was talking to some students the other day and they said, 'Oh, you've forgotten something' and I said 'Oh yes, I have got a good reason to forget. I am brain damaged.' And they said, 'Yeah!' I said, 'Yes, look, I've got a dent in my head to prove it!' and then they looked a bit shocked, So I said, 'Yes, I've had brain surgery.' And at that point they don't know if you're joking or not.

Turning to books

Several people talked about books that they felt had helped with their recovery. Some of these supplemented the information on subarachnoid haemorrhage they had been given in hospital. Tania, for example, read 'loads of books about brain haemorrhages'. Learning about other people's experiences meant she didn't feel alone with what had happened to her. She also suggested it could be helpful if relatives read some of the titles.

Reading about other kinds of illness or injury could also be helpful. Following a below-the-knee amputation, Jane Grant (2006) also turned to reading narratives of illness, leading her to ask: 'Should professionals "prescribe" narratives?' as she found this had many benefits during an extremely traumatic time:

Reading narratives of trauma, illness, loss, provided insight, inspiration, enjoyment and epiphany during an acutely traumatic period. I could begin to make sense of my feelings and discover myself in relation to others who'd been in similar positions before me. I wasn't alone.

(Grant 2006)

Sandra and Andrew also read widely. Sandra found that books played an important part in helping her to clarify the new directions in her life that she was seeking:

> I read lots of books . . . books on 'how to' . . . I think I kind of left myself to stumble upon things, because I didn't really know what direction to go in . . . and I would go into a shop and a book would get my attention and I would think – that's the book I need today. And I would find a piece in it that comforted me or reassured me or gave me a sense of purpose or a direction to go in, and that seemed to be enough.

Andrew too turned to self-help books, but he also found support in reading books about spirituality. As he says: 'There were strange encouragements out of all sorts of things that I read . . . I don't know if other people have had any similar experiences or felt an urge to read any of these things.'

So reading seems to have helped and supported people in many different ways – lessening their sense of isolation, reassuring them that others have been through this experience, offering ideas about how to cope with things like depression, and providing guidance about making life changes.

14

CHANGED LIVES

This is the final chapter, but for many their journey of recovery continues – sometimes over many years. Here, survivors take stock, reflect on their experiences and talk about how their lives have changed – in the way they see the world and their place in it. The journey of recovery is often neither easy nor straightforward. There can be persisting deficits or disabilities and adjusting to these can be difficult (Larner 2005). I hope, however, that the last two chapters show that the journey of recovery can ultimately result in positive changes along the way. This is certainly a view espoused by Trevor Powell:

> People often find spiritual meaning and a change in their values after the experience of a brain injury. It slows people down, stops people racing in life and allows more time for thoughtful contemplation. It raises questions about the meaning of life and what is and is not important. It changes people's views of themselves and their own vulnerability and mortality. Greater emphasis is often placed on relationships, real friends and closeness to family members . . . some people say that they have become kinder, their values have changed, they appreciate their life more and have greater tolerance of the vulnerabilities of others.
>
> (Powell 2004: 201)

A life-changing experience

A positive experience

Survivors are frequently aware that the haemorrhage had been a life-changing event. Vernon described it as 'a huge life-changing

219

experience'. Andrew also felt he had changed: 'I don't know if people would say I've changed, but I feel in myself I have changed and I'm conscious of wanting to make a change.'

When Gillen (2005) interviewed a group of stroke survivors, nearly two-thirds were able to identify positive consequences, including personal growth, greater health awareness and increased social relationships. Janet echoed this when she wrote: 'I look on the whole experience as a very positive one and feel that good things have come out of it.' For someone like Megan, having a brain haemorrhage was not only life-changing but also offered the opportunity for learning from the experience:

> I think we're the product of our experience, aren't we? So whatever experience you have, hopefully you'll do something with it – do something useful with it. I think life is the learning curve – and you're never the same, because you've got another string to your bow, haven't you? You've got this other new experience you can share with people . . . I can understand how difficult it is to suddenly find your life's got to change dramatically . . . but yes, we do change, it does change you.

With a life-threatening episode such as subarachnoid haemorrhage, even when recovery has been relatively straightforward, 'for many people such a traumatic event will divide into life before and life after' (Tschudin 1997: 75). Rosie's haemorrhage was three and a half years ago so she says: 'That's why I say I'm three and half years! It's a whole new life. A new me!' And for Sandra it had 'felt like being reborn'.

A second chance

Having survived a brain haemorrhage it can feel like being given 'a second chance' (Hop *et al.* 1998: 803). This was how Lesley saw it:

> I feel – you know, the biblical phrase 'the scales have fallen from my eyes' – as if I've been offered an insight into a different way of being . . . [it] offered me a different way of seeing myself in the world and seeing the world. . . . I feel as if I've been given another chance, that I've been offered an

opportunity to see life differently and I want to grab it with both hands and not slide into a kind of middle-aged mediocrity.

The other way in which people described this opportunity was that the haemorrhage had acted as a 'wake-up call'. As Sandra explained:

It's been a real journey for me and I couldn't have begun it without having what I call a real kick up the backside . . . I don't regret one second of any of it . . . it was such a wake-up call and I really needed it.

Things could have been worse

Feeling that life has changed for the better may depend on whether someone has made a reasonably good recovery and survivors were sometimes aware that, despite continuing difficulties, the outcome could have been worse. Nochi describes this as 'the self better than others' as survivors of brain injury 'contrasted the present self with comparable images that looked worse' (2000: 1797). Rosie realises she could have been left with more significant disabilities:

I've always looked on it as a positive experience. All very well for me to say that because I'm not left with any deficit. When I saw my consultant three or four months after I'd had the aneurysm, he said, 'How are you doing?' and I said, 'Absolutely fine. Wonderful. Am I unusual in recovering so completely?' He said, 'Yes, I saw a chap this morning who had the same thing as you on the same day and he's not even able to speak.' And that puts it all into perspective.

Lesley was also aware that the outcomes could have been very different so was able to put her continuing difficulties into perspective:

I am so lucky. I could be lying in a hospital bed being turned every two hours and somebody feeding me and somebody mopping up the other end. So – I've had a brain haemorrhage; I've had it and I'm going to live my life every day to the best of

221

my ability even though I might say the wrong words, trip up over my words, trip up over my feet!

Growth through trauma

Chapter 4 described the traumatic aspects of surviving a brain haemorrhage, but there is growing evidence that trauma can also lead to positive changes in people's lives – to 'post-traumatic growth (Linley and Joseph 2002), or to put it another way, 'there's no gain without pain':

> We suggest that post-traumatic growth may be experi-
> enced simultaneously to post traumatic stress symptoms . . .
> the experience of growth is not the same as the absence of
> distress, but that both might co-exist.
>
> (Linley and Joseph 2002: 16)

David is making a good recovery but, as he recalls, things weren't always that positive and life was often stressful and difficult:

> My main thing was, would I be normal again because I felt
> abnormal. I felt as if I was disabled in some way because of the
> operation I'd had and because I was so weak. I had no strength
> . . . I ran the Great North Run two weeks before this happened
> . . . from running the Great North Run in one hour 45 minutes to
> not being able to walk ten paces is quite a big thing to under-
> stand. As far as I was concerned my whole life had finished. I
> couldn't work, I couldn't run. I was moody and constantly tired
> and constantly being sick . . . I'd lost everything I wanted.

As he went on to say: 'Because it takes so long to actually get better, we have an awful lot of spare time to reflect. I know I certainly have – on my past and my future.' Post-traumatic growth can go hand in hand with post-traumatic stress, but 'is unlikely in the immediate aftermath of trauma but rather arises as a result of the rumination and restructuring that takes place in the weeks, months and even years following the trauma' (Linley and Joseph 2002: 16). As Patsy has found:

I always say, my life will never be the same as it was before. Socially, physically, my life has changed; the fact that I can't work in any paid employment any more; I can't do all the things that I want to do . . . so there are a lot of things. Your life does change, doesn't it? Perhaps as we knew it, for the better . . . You are learning to adapt to this new way of life. For some of us it can be a better way of life and you've got to hope that it is.

Searching for meaning

Viktor Frankl suggests that 'we can discover the meaning in life . . . by the attitude we take towards unavoidable suffering' (1959: 133). When people are going through a health crisis and looking for meaning:

> A search for meaning is reflected in questions such as 'Why did it happen?' 'What impact has it had?' 'What does my life mean now?' A search for meaning can be understood in terms of a search for causality and a search to understand the implications.
>
> (Ogden 2000: 62)

Following a brain haemorrhage, survivors can have many questions. As Robert McCrum writes about the aftermath of his haemorrhagic stroke:

> A stroke will open up an almost unending vista of questions about yourself and your significance . . . And yet the question Why? continues to hover over almost every day of your life, though before you can get to the Why? you have to ask yourself What? What was it that I went through? What exactly is its significance? What does it mean? These are the questions which bring us inexorably back to Why?
>
> (McCrum 1998: 215–16)

Although there are some known risk factors for subarachnoid haemorrhage, our understanding of why aneurysms develop and why they sometimes rupture is incomplete. However, this doesn't stop people wondering why this has happened (or others asking them for an explanation). The survivor's search to understand the meaning of their haemorrhage can lead them to question why it happened. For Robert McCrum, this search for 'Why?', although it didn't produce any answers, led him to conclude that there was a kind of meaning to what happened to him:

> In my case, since the doctors have failed to find a reliable explanation for my stroke, I like to think that I was profoundly lucky. If there is a God, he is remote, detached and impressively hands-off. I am inclined to say that at first I didn't think there was anyone out there for me, and then that I had been cruelly punished without reason, and yet, finally, that there was an odd kind of purpose to everything that happened.
>
> (McCrum 1998: 216)

When I asked the survivors why they thought their haemorrhage had occurred, some people said that they'd never really thought about that. Others though put it down to chance, fate or bad luck ('shit happens and you move on' as Karen-Ann said). They didn't feel that they were to blame or that they had somehow caused the haemorrhage. In other words, they could accept that what happened had been beyond their control. For the majority of survivors, their haemorrhage had resulted from a ruptured aneurysm, but for someone like Andrew, where no aneurysm was found, the search for 'Why?' can continue:

> The question mark would be there all the time and I couldn't quite understand what had happened because they couldn't find anything . . . I think I questioned my wife to the nth degree . . . I think I drove her up the wall . . . it left me with a question which it still leaves me with to this day.

Although researchers have concluded that stressful life events do not constitute a risk factor for subarachnoid haemorrhage (Powell *et al.* 2002: 779), some people still believed that stress had been a contributory factor. Sandra talked about how 'very serious stress . . . had built up to that particular day and that's why my head exploded'. Christine, who had a very demanding job, afterwards 'spent a lot of time thinking, blaming myself. Because I'd put so much effort into this job'. If stress may not, in fact, have played a part, what does perhaps matter is that, as a result, people decided to adopt a less stressful lifestyle. Perhaps this was also a way in which they could find meaning in what had happened – in the sense that the haemorrhage had served some purpose. This was what Patsy felt:

> I do think to myself, perhaps I was meant to have the haemorrhage for a reason. Perhaps out of this haemorrhage, something else is happening to my life . . . I've had the haemorrhage, I have survived it, so you've got to make something from it, haven't you?

A changed outlook on life

Survivors of trauma often find their philosophy of life has altered. This may involve shifting their priorities, having a fresh appreciation of each day and realising that life is finite (Linley and Joseph 2002).

Deciding what really matters

A subarachnoid haemorrhage can lead to people reviewing their priorities and deciding what really matters to them now. This can involve making actual changes in the way they live or simply having a different outlook on life. In Lauren's words 'It affects your values.' And as Janice has found:

> I think providing it doesn't kill you, it does you the world of good! Because I have found that emotionally, this makes you realise what is important and what isn't – more especially that we fret and worry about superficial things that don't really matter. It's done me the world of good in that respect, in that it's focused my mind on things that do really matter.

Rosie's priorities have also changed, and she no longer wants to devote time and energy to things which previously mattered:

> My priorities completely changed . . . things that were important then, just don't matter now . . . I was involved with the residents association and we'd be fighting for people who didn't want next door to build a garage and don't like that fence over there.

It's not important! I should be dead now and I'm not and that's what's important. I'm alive now and I've got to make the best that I can with the physical abilities I've been left with. I really don't care if next door paints her house blue – it's her house!

The work–life balance can shift as people find that their priorities have changed and they will not resume their previous lifestyle (Powell *et al.* 2002: 779). As Wendy concluded, the haemorrhage has made her rethink her lifestyle – and decide that housework isn't really important:

[It's] brought me much closer to my husband and family. It's made me much less busy at work . . . now I'm not prepared to keep offering to take on extra work. I've changed my work–life balance and my home life is much more important to me than my work . . . it might have been difficult to know if I had it the right way round before. My outlook on life has certainly changed . . . It's been a very long hard road though and thinking actually what is important in life and what do I want from life. Does it matter if I haven't dusted the house for three weeks? Not really, and if you've got friends coming round that comment on it, then they'll have to get the duster out.

So, as Wendy says, family matters more, echoed by Tania who commented that 'rediscovering family and friends in a new light has been a big life-changer'. Others have found that 'social relationships were appreciated more than before' (Hop *et al.* 1998: 803).

Slowing down

Moving out of the fast lane and enjoying a gentler pace of life can be a positive choice. Perhaps the enforced 'leisure' in the early stages of recovery can give someone a taste of a more relaxed lifestyle. As Christine said of her first year of recovery: 'There was a sort of slowness to life which is nice.' Veronica too has adjusted to a different lifestyle during her recovery: 'I've learned to take life at a slower pace. I'm the sort of person that rushes from A to B all the time. I think I've learned to pace myself.'

Deciding to slow down and relax more may be because people are working fewer hours or because they have chosen to or been forced to retire early (Ogden *et al.* 1997; see also Chapter 12). Karen was used to juggling her roles of mother, wife and worker, but although she still hopes to perhaps return to work in the future, she says:

> I think I made the choice actually to not juggle quite so many balls any more. I don't know whether that was a conscious choice or whether that's the way I am now . . . I don't want to be fast and running about; I'm a bit more relaxed I suppose.

Slowing down could also mean becoming more patient. Having been a successful chef before his haemorrhage, David was used to working at a very rapid pace: 'Whereas before I used to [say] "Now! Now! Now!" it's now "Okay, I'll do it in a minute, sort of thing".'

Noticing 'things of nature'

People often turn instinctively to nature, to the outdoors, when looking for peace and relaxation, so it was not surprising that several survivors noticed their increased awareness of the natural world. As John wrote, since his haemorrhage he is 'more aware of a beautiful day, "hello birds, hello trees"'. Pam also experienced this heightened appreciation:

> I think after having the haemorrhage it made me appreciate little things . . . just little things like watching a row of ants carting bits of soil to make their nest and thinking – your life is as precious to you as mine is to me . . . just fascinating.

Maybe we have yet to discover a link between recovery from sub-arachnoid haemorrhage and an interest in insect life, as Vernon also said:

> Nature for me was a load of rubbish. I wasn't interested in it and even though I was brought up in the countryside I didn't care about the minute details of life, but now, I'm interested. I could sit down and watch a fly buzz about!

While survivors were sometimes engaged in rethinking their lives overall, perhaps the enforced time and space offering opportunities for contemplation also presented the chance to notice the otherwise unremarked on and unnoticed. Spending time with what she described as 'things of nature', Janice feels that this has been an important part of her recovery:

> I sit here and I look at this lovely garden . . . pond gazing is a very good relaxer; I just sit there and I watch my tadpoles swimming around, and the frogs and newts and fish . . . the wind blowing in the trees, the waves, the sea coming in . . . things like that are a natural relaxer . . . that is what heals me.

Realising life is finite

When survivors realise that their haemorrhage had been life threatening and that 50 per cent do not survive the haemorrhage, this may heighten their awareness that death can occur at any time and that life is not limited. It's a case of seize the day – *carpe diem* – or 'seize the carp' as Robert McCrum describes it (1998: 191). And as Lauren had found:

> You think about the amount of time you might have left and what you're going to do with it . . . I think the close scrape with death has caused me to realise where I need to make even more changes to bring about a happier and more peaceful existence.

The reminder that life is finite can act as a catalyst, with survivors wanting to hold on to that awareness and make the most of the remaining years. For Lesley this was:

> another kind of knock on the door to say, come on, life is not endless, make the most of it! It's like a kind of warning – get going! It's a real sort of awakener that there's less time left . . . and I don't want to look back in ten or 15 years and say 'I wish I'd made more of what I can do!'

After Sandra's second haemorrhage within a year, she realised that the present was what mattered; perhaps 'seize the day' could also mean seizing control of one's life:

That event made me sit up and realise that now is the only
thing that matters – the only thing that's real is now! I used to
believe that 'one day' this would happen and 'one day' that
would happen and 'if only this will happen, then that will
happen' [but] it's how I'm conducting myself now; that's all that
counts.

At home recovering from his haemorrhage, Brian spent time
with his elderly father and other relatives, looking at family photos
and finding out about his family's history. As he says, this is the
kind of thing you can keep putting off, but then realised that with
elderly relatives it can be too late: 'Actually you've only got a
certain amount of time . . . you need to have a near-death experience to actually improve your life and do the interesting things you
wouldn't normally do.' For Graham too, his haemorrhage led him
to realise the importance of not procrastinating:

It's made me really appreciate just how precious life is. It alters
your whole perspective on it and I don't say I'm going to do this
in ten years' time. If you can, do it now, because you don't
know what's around the corner.

With this focus on the present, there can also be a heightened
appreciation of each day. As Christine explained: 'I don't think too
far down the road . . . I just think, no, enjoy today.' And Pam sees
the greatest gain as being the joy of having survived and her
appreciation of life:

I think before, I took life for granted. I'd get up, I'd go to work, I
brought up my daughter, I'd walk the dogs. But now, everything
is a pleasure to do – even in the puddles and the biting wind.
Even if I fall and I'm dirty and I'm cold, I'll say 'Yeah, you're
alive!'

Realising that life is finite may also mean that survivors can find
death and dying less fearful, as Veronica said:

At one time I'd have been terrified of dying . . . But I think
because I know that I have been very close to dying, I'm now

more accepting of dying. I'm not saying I'm ready to die but I'm not frightened of dying.

Spirituality and religion

Coping strategies can include finding comfort in religion or spiritual beliefs and praying or meditating (Carver 1997). My topic guide for the interviews included the question: 'Since your bleed, would you consider yourself religious or spiritual?' As Trevor Powell also suggests: 'People often find spiritual meaning . . . after a brain injury' (2004: 191). Terms like 'religious' or 'spiritual' are not easily defined (particularly in the latter case), but people usually talked about religion in terms of a set of beliefs (e.g. a belief in God) and practices (e.g. praying). For Andrew, Christianity has played an important part in his recovery. Having previously been a practising Christian, but having moved away from the Church, he now found that his 'relationship with God [was] rekindled [and] opened up the Christian life again'. Rosie too had ceased to be a practising Christian, but after her haemorrhage was still able to draw on her religious beliefs:

> I've always been a Christian, but for a long long time not a practising Christian . . . so I lost faith in Christians but not in my God, or that God I perceive Him to be. And I just think perhaps He gave me a lot of peace.

Although other survivors talked more about spirituality, this wasn't always necessarily seen as being separate from religious beliefs. Lauren described how significant pre-haemorrhage losses had led her:

> to a kind of spiritual place – not deeply religious, but spiritual . . . when I realised I was up against something that my brain couldn't handle I'd just say 'Please God!' And hand it over . . . because that has been so helpful, it's probably deepened my sense of spirituality around the whole thing.

Surviving a life-threatening event, having 'the chance to stare death in the face', as Lesley described it, had also made her more open to exploring spirituality:

[It] created in me a great awareness of my feelings about spirituality . . . I suppose I've always had a sense of the outdoors as being my cathedral and it's interesting that I was reading not so long ago about the improved speed in healing if people can see greenery . . . there is something about that that provides comfort and healing . . . I find it really hard to articulate this – something about just feeling closer to a sense of spirituality? I'm open, much more open to the possibilities of a more spiritual way of being and I use that in my [psychotherapy] work quite a lot now . . . so, yes, perhaps I am more spiritual.

Perhaps what Lesley is struggling to articulate is reflected in the US National Cancer Institute's (2007) definition of spirituality as 'having to do with deep, often religious feelings and beliefs, including a person's sense of peace, purpose, connection to others and beliefs about the meaning of life'. Although Tania does not ascribe her feelings and experiences to any formal religious beliefs, she does emphasise not only her joyfulness but her connection to other people:

Not a formal belief thing or a certain religion, no. But I feel feelings that maybe some people I could imagine ascribing to a religious feeling but I'm just very joyful about life and ecstatic to be back at work . . . and getting real joy out of small things and I'm so close to my family and friends now.

A changed view of the self

Viktor Frankl suggests that 'when we are no longer able to change a situation . . . we are challenged to change ourselves' (1959: 135). There is no doubt that having a brain haemorrhage changes many people's lives – but does it change them as a person? Like others who have been through a traumatic event, survivors may find their view of themselves has changed in some ways. They may feel they have become stronger and more resilient, but may also become more accepting of any limitations and vulnerabilities they are now living with (Linley and Joseph 2002).

Chapter 13 discussed how survivors may become stronger and more resilient when they realise that they have the determination and strength to help themselves recover. As Wendy said: 'I probably am a stronger person than I realised and there was this strong sense that I wanted to get my life back.' On the whole Roy has made a good recovery, but still needs practical help sometimes. The haemorrhage has yielded gains and losses to his sense of self: 'I would like to be the physical person I was, but the emotional person I am now.' His physical self has changed in ways he finds difficult, but he is having to accept his limitations and vulnerabilities – the loss of a physically independent self.

Same person – but different

When I asked the survivors whether they felt they had changed in any way as a result of their experiences, they were sometimes puzzled or uncertain about how to reply. Am I the same person as before or am I different? Veronica was thinking aloud:

> I'm different. I feel different . . . I won't say I feel worse than I felt before, but it's different, it's a different feeling . . . I haven't changed but I have changed! So although I'm the same person, I'm a different person. I can't really put it into words. I don't think I'm ever going to be the same person that I was before [the haemorrhage] but I'm very close to that person . . . I'm very nearly there.

So there is a sense that the former self – the pre-haemorrhage self – can be reclaimed but alongside this there are changes. As Lauren explained: 'I think I'm largely back to, in many respects, as I was – but changed. I'm just a different person now. I've got a different view of the world.'

The reasons why someone may feel they have changed – that they are now, to some extent a different person – can also be difficult for someone to understand. Have they become a different person because of their brain injury or have they changed because of their enforced lifestyle change? Scott who had a haemorrhagic stroke and developed hydrocephalus and epilepsy wonders if both play a part:

> I don't want to use the phrase 'a completely different person', because I'm not . . . I have changed considerably, but whether

it's because of the neurological side of it or the whole life change. I think if you were to take somebody – anybody – and completely change their life, then they would change as a person, but we've got the added complication of our brains having had a little stir.

A year after her haemorrhage which left her with severe cognitive difficulties, Heather is struggling to understand this:

So many people have said to me that I have changed since [the haemorrhage] and I can't see that because I still only see me and I'm still here and the same person. But obviously my actions and my personality have changed, so that's a bit weird really; it feels a bit spooky! Because you can't remember what you were like before, so you can't try and be more like that.

The grown self

Nochi coins this phrase when writing about how people coping with traumatic brain injury described their experiences: 'the experience of TBI [traumatic brain injury] had contributed at least a certain positive characteristic to the scenario of their lives' (2000: 1798). These positives included having greater insight into themselves and greater understanding and empathy for other people. It would hardly be surprising if the experience of a sudden illness and lengthy recovery did not change people in some ways. People sometimes expressed this in terms of personal qualities – empathy for others, for example. At other times they were perhaps talking about generally becoming more 'emotionally literate' (Orbach 1999) – more aware of and in touch with their feelings:

I've learned more about what I am as a person and it gives you more insight into how you tick, how you cope with things.

(Andrew)

And now I do feel emotions a lot more. I'm aware of my emotions and what they might mean. They've changed a lot – my emotions – because before, I'd blocked all my emotions out and because I was working in the building trade as well . . . I've

233

got a different outlook on relationships . . . I've got more understanding, I think, of people.

(Vernon)

Growing up and growing through?

Tania was 31 at the time of her haemorrhage and now, as she says: 'I'm definitely more grown up; a definite kind of change in that phase of my life before and now this phase and I'm more grown up and organised.' This changed and more grown-up self can also be welcomed, as Rosie found: 'I think I probably used to make an idiot of myself. I've grown up. I've calmed down and I like myself a lot better. I like the way I am now.'

If survivors saw these changes in themselves, sometimes the haemorrhage could lead to someone gaining a clearer sense of themselves, of their identity, for the first time. As Sandra explains:

> [The haemorrhage] allowed me to recognise myself. It's given me an identity I didn't know I had. I think it started with the care of all the medical staff, the ambulance staff. They're fantastic people and they made me acknowledge myself . . . they were working to save *me* . . . I had to acknowledge that that's what they were working for.

A word of caution, however – change isn't compulsory. When asked if he felt he had changed since his haemorrhage, John's response was simply: 'Would that that were so.'

Are you lucky?

I asked survivors whether they ever felt that they were lucky to have had a brain haemorrhage. This might seem a strange question but I wanted to ask people because so many had said this to me and, as I rightly guessed, others had been told that too. Survivors were often unsure about whether they did feel 'lucky':

> When you look at the statistics and you see that 50 per cent don't make it . . . I don't know if lucky is the word. I suppose I've been given an insight into things that other people wouldn't necessarily gain.

(Andrew)

I class myself as lucky, I think . . . I could have been luckier had
it not happened at all [but] the crying's over with; you've just got
to pick yourself up, dust yourself off and crack on with life. I
think, yes, I am lucky.

(David)

Feeling lucky or being grateful that you're alive – it may not
always seem like that and can be particularly difficult when, like
Karen, recovery sometimes feels such an uphill struggle:

I'd say I did have a stage of being grateful that I was alive and
then when I had the days when I just had tears and I felt real
frustration, I wasn't bloody grateful! I'd think, no, I'm not
grateful for having to put up with this! I shouldn't have to be
grateful and I wasn't . . . There have been times when I've
really got to rock bottom and wondered why I'd bothered to
survive.

Luck seems to have more than one meaning here. Survivors may
indeed feel lucky in the sense that they were fortunate to still be
alive. On the other hand, they may not feel so lucky when, as Karen
describes, recovery can be slow, difficult and such hard work.

Gains and losses

There are many losses associated with having a brain haemorrhage.
Some are immediate though sometimes temporary, while others
may be longer lasting. Previous chapters have already touched on
some of these losses relating to physical difficulties, emotional
problems and cognitive impairments. But as this chapter also
discusses, there can be gains – a newly discovered appreciation of
life itself, a reordering of priorities, for example. For many people
the haemorrhage will bring both losses and gains in its wake. When
Pam had a haemorrhagic stroke, the potential losses at first were
many – 'I thought I'd lost my job! I'd lost my [counselling] course
. . . you're not sure whether your husband or partner's going to stay
with you.' But as she found, the gains have outweighed the losses
'because what's been lost in one area has been made up in other
areas . . . four years down the line I've lost nothing. I've gained
from it'.

One year after a haemorrhage, the actress Jane Lapotaire described her losses: 'the loss of my work, the loss of several friends, the loss of the world I knew and the loss of confidence and trust in myself' (2003: 258). However, on the final page of her book she writes: 'It has given me a better life. I don't have as much of lots of the things I had before, but I have more of what I never had. As they say in the theatre, less is more. What a paradox.'

At the beginning – and sometimes for months or even years – there are many losses, but gradually over time the experience of recovery can offer gains as well. Vernon, who left hospital with significant disabilities, looks back:

> I don't feel like I've lost so much now, but initially I felt like I'd lost more. There's lots and lots of losses that I initially felt . . . obviously my mind – there's things like memory . . . function of my body. I lost friends . . . there's so many losses, really. But I've also gained a lot as well. I've gained a lot of insight into life and I've gained a lot of understanding, I think, of myself.

The losses which people sustain can be experienced as a bereavement, with a period of mourning (Hager and Ziegler 1998, cited in Scott 2006; Jarvis 2002). In her interviews with people 14 to 18 months after their haemorrhage, Jarvis described 'a sense of a grieving process and grief for the previous self' and what one of her interviewees described as 'a kind of grief for my former activities' (Jarvis 2002: 1435).

Because there are often lengthy timescales of recovery, for some people this can feel like lost time and the loss of 'what might have been'. Although Lauren realises she has gained much from her experience, as she says:

> I do get moments when I feel bereaved . . . I think I've lost a bit of a chunk of my life from what might have [been]. I think the past two years have been very much focused around recovery, rather than actually maybe doing other things or meeting other people.

Wendy too can see many gains from her recent experiences, but like Lauren she was also mourning lost time:

I feel I've lost a part of my life, particularly with . . . the depression that came as a result of it . . . Because there are weeks or months of my life where I think I'm just existing and not living, and you're getting through because you have to get through and you're not going to get that time again, in particular with my daughter and so many things she's been going through just as a teenager.

For Christine, cognitive difficulties have continued to some extent, and this for her is a loss:

I'm frustrated that my brain doesn't work like it used to and I do feel that I always had a brightish brain and I just feel that it doesn't work as well as it used to . . . I can't pinpoint what doesn't work particularly, because I can still do crosswords and Sudoku, so that seems to work, you know? But there's certainly something that doesn't . . . and that I find a loss.

But she is clear that these losses are set against gains:

I've got no sense of loss about my job now; that was just something I did. I get more reward from what I'm doing now, although it's considerably less money . . . it's much more rewarding. And again [I've] slowed down, definitely, which is nice.

Getting back to normal?

Getting back to normal varies from person to person:

It can take many months following a subarachnoid haemorrhage to feel that life is getting back to 'normal' and people often ask if they will ever be the same again. This is a very difficult question to answer as everyone's recovery is different.
(Brain and Spine Foundation 2005b: 16)

From the professionals' perspective 'the desirable clinical outcome is typically a resumption of "life as normal"' (Powell *et al.* 2002),

237

but these researchers also went on to say that 'the road to recovery need not necessarily focus on promoting resumption of prior or even "normal" patterns of activity' (Powell *et al.* 2004: 1124). As with being told 'you've been lucky', the phrase 'getting back to normal' seems to carry several different messages. For survivors, 'getting back to normal' can mean being able to walk down the road, doing the shopping, reading a book, going back to work – aspects of daily life which we generally take for granted. Something that Shirley wrote, entitled 'Normal', offers yet another perspective:

> I find myself writing this down as it is the only way I think that people will understand. For the last eighteen months, ever since my brain haemorrhage, I have continually used the phrase 'when I am back to normal'. As the improvement in both my mental and physical abilities seems now to have reached a plateau, I think I am at the stage of accepting that yes, I am back to normal. *But normal is not what it was before.* [italics added]

If life after a brain haemorrhage is different, it can still be normal, can't it? Perhaps this is also about being able to resume a more 'ordinary' life or lifestyle? A fair chunk of this book is about the 'ordinary', the day to day. For someone who has not been through recovery from a brain haemorrhage, reading about shopping, driving, enjoying books and watching television may come across as boring or banal at times. But when, for the survivor, these elements of daily life are suddenly not possible (for a time at least) then they are certainly neither boring nor banal.

Afterword

During my recovery, I came across a poem with the title 'Jigsaw'. Although not specifically addressing the subject of brain haemorrhage, some survivors have described their recovery as like piecing together a jigsaw so some lines from this poem seem an appropriate point with which to end:

> Don't dwell on the gaps
> On what's missing
> What's there makes some sense

Even if it's incomplete
Celebrate what has been connected

. . .

Nothing can be forced
Nothing can be rushed

(Ward 2001)

APPENDIX A

Table of participating survivors: interviews and written accounts

Name	Date of SAH(s)	Age at time of SAH(s)
Andrew	November 2004	45
Brian	January 2006	42
Christine	November 1999	43
David	October 2005	40
Faith	June 1987	55
Graham	December 1997	54
Heather	May 2005	33
James	October 2001	68
Jan	December 2003	54
Janet*	September 2005	45
Janice	1983 and October 2005	54
Jessica	September 2002	23
John*	June 2002	58
Karen	July 2005	42
Karen-Ann	May 2002	40
Kaz	May 1991	28
Lauren	4 July 2004	48
Lesley	September 2002	51
Megan	July 2005	58
Pam	1972 and February 2002	50
Patsy	January 2005	48
Rosie	November 2002	44
Roy	February 2003	56
Sandra	July 1994 and	40
	April 1995	41
Scott	May 2003	35
Shirley*	February 2005	46
Tania	December 2003	31
Vernon	July 1998	28
Veronica	October 2003	58
Wendy	November 2002	42

* Written contribution

APPENDIX B

USEFUL ORGANISATIONS

Brain and Spine Foundation
7 Winchester House
Cranmer Road
London SW9 6EJ
Helpline: 0808 808 1000

Brain and Spine Injury Charity (BASIC)
The Neurocare Centre
554 Eccles New Road
Salford M5 5AP
Helpline: 0870 750 0000

Brain Aneurysm Foundation
269 Hanover Street, Building 3
Hanover
MA 02339
USA
Tel: (from UK) 001 781 826 5556

Different Strokes
Different Strokes Central Services
9 Canon Harnett Court
Wolverton Mill
Milton Keynes MK12 5NF
Tel: 0845 130 7172
Email: info@differentstrokes.co.uk

Epilepsy Action (British Epilepsy Association)
New Anstey House
Gate Way Drive
Yeadon
Leeds LS18 7XY
Tel: 0113 210 8800
Helpline: 0808 800 5050

Headway
4 King Edward Court
King Edward Street
Nottingham NG1 1EW
Tel: 0115 924 0800
Helpline: 0808 800 2244

National Society for Epilepsy
Chesham Lane
Chalfont St Peter
Gerrards Cross
Buckinghamshire SL9 ORJ
Tel: 01494 601 300
Helpline: 01494 601 400

Stroke Association
Stroke House
240 City Road
London EC1V 2PR
Tel: 0207 566 0300
Helpline: 0845 3033 100

Val Hennessy Trust
8 Queen Victoria Road
Coventry CV1 3JH
Tel: 02476 634 601

APPENDIX C

SUPPORT GROUPS

Edinburgh
Brain Aneurysm Self-Help (BASH)
Tel: 0131 337 8663 / 0131 467 2707

Newcastle
Subarachnoid Haemorrhage Support Group for Patients and Carers
Neuroradiology Department
Newcastle General Hospital
Newcastle NE4 6BE
Tel: 0191 256 3347 / 0191 256 3395

Nottingham
Cerebral Aneurysm Support Group
Tel: 07791 763537
Email: casg2005@btinternet.com

Salford / Greater Manchester
BASIC SAH Support Group
Tel: 0870 750 000
Email: enquiries@basiccharity.org.uk

Southampton / Wessex
Subarachnoid Haemorrhage and Cerebral Aneurysm Support Group
Wessex Neurological Centre
Southampton General Hospital
Tremona Road
Southampton SO16 6YD
Tel: 023 8079 8428

APPENDIX D

GLOSSARY OF TERMS

aneurysm   A balloon-like swelling in the wall of an artery caused by disease or an inherited deficiency.

angiogram   X-ray examination of blood vessels.

aphasia   Language disorder arising from damage to areas of the brain that control understanding and expression of spoken and written language; also called dysphasia.

arachnoid   The middle of the three membranes covering the brain and spinal cord.

artery   A blood vessel carrying blood away from the heart.

catheter   A flexible tube for insertion into a narrow opening so that fluids may be introduced or removed.

cerebral angiogram   An investigation using X-ray which looks at the blood vessels in the brain, used to help find the cause of the subarachnoid haemorrhage.

cerebro-spinal fluid (CSF)   The clear watery fluid that surrounds and protects the brain and spinal cord.

clipping   The placing of a metal or plastic clip across an aneurysm in order to secure it.

cognitive function   All the normal processes associated with our thoughts and mental processes.

coiling   The placing of metal coils within an aneurysm in order to secure it.

computerised tomography (CT)   An X-ray system which uses computers to provide a series of cross-sectional pictures of the body.

dysarthria   A speech impairment affecting voice production, articulation, resonance and intonation.

dysphasia   See aphasia.

embolisation   Alternative term for coiling (see above).

epilepsy   Disorder of the brain usually characterised by recurrent attacks of unconsciousness (fits or seizures).

haemorrhage   The escape of blood from a ruptured blood vessel, externally or internally.

hydrocephalus   An abnormal increase in the amount of cerebro-spinal fluid within the cavities of the brain.

lumbar puncture   A procedure in which cerebro-spinal fluid is extracted for diagnostic purposes by means of a hollow needle inserted into the sub-arachnoid space in the region of the lower back.

membrane   A thin layer of tissue surrounding an organ or tissue, lining a cavity or separating structures or cavities.

magnetic resonance imaging (MRI)   A type of scan which makes use of magnetic fields and radio waves to provide images of the internal structure of the body.

neurological   Refers to conditions occurring in the nervous system including the brain, spine and all the peripheral nerves.

neurosurgeon   A specialist doctor within neurosurgery who treats patients following a subarachnoid haemorrhage.

occupational therapy   Treatment that uses specific activities to help people whose physical and particularly movement capabilities have been damaged to recover what skills they can to help them lead as normal and independent a life as possible.

physiotherapy   Treatment that uses physical methods to promote healing, including the use of light, heat, electric current massage, manipulation and exercise.

scan   The examination of the body or part of the body, such as the brain, using CT or MRI (see above).

shunt   A tube which is passed from the inside of the brain to the abdominal cavity to drain the cerebro-spinal fluid when the normal route is blocked.

speech therapy   Treatment that helps patients whose speech has been affected to speak clearly again.

stroke   A sudden attack of weakness affecting one side of the body resulting from an interruption to the flow of blood to the brain.

subarachnoid haemorrhage (SAH)   A sudden leakage of blood across the base of the brain.

vasospasm   Narrowing of the arteries within the brain, potentially restricting the blood flow.

X-ray contrast   A substance (sometimes called a dye) injected to show up the difference between different types of tissue.

Sources: Brain and Spine Foundation (1998, 2002); Foulkes (2004).

REFERENCES

Al-Shahi, R., White, P.M., Davenport, R.J. and Lindsay. K.W. (2006) 'Subarachnoid haemorrhage: clinical review', *British Medical Journal*, 333: 235–40.

Anthony, W.A. (1993) 'Recovery from mental illness: the guiding vision of the mental health service system in the 1990s', *Psychosocial Rehabilitation*, 16(4): 11–23.

BBC (2004) 'Your Life in Their Hands': Programme 1; transmitted 8 March.

Beristain, X., Gaviria, M., Dujovny, M., El-Bary, T.H.A., Stark, J.L. and Ausman, J.I. (1996) 'Evaluation of outcome after incracranial aneurysm surgery: the neuropsychiatric approach', *Surgical Neurology*, 45: 422–9.

Blastland, M., Vickers, N. and Happé, F. (2007) 'In sickness and in hope', *Prospect*, 138: 48–51.

British Medical Journal (BMJ, 2002) 'From patients to end users', Editorial, *British Medical Journal*, 424: 555–6.

Boss, P. (2006) *Loss, Trauma and Resilience: Therapeutic Work with Ambiguous Loss*. New York/London: Norton.

Brain and Spine Foundation (1998) *Speech, Language and Communication Difficulties*. London: Brain and Spine Foundation.

Brain and Spine Foundation (2002) *Sub-Arachnoid Haemorrhage: A Guide for Patients and Carers*. London: Brain and Spine Foundation.

Brain and Spine Foundation (2005a) *Coiling of Brain Aneurysms: A Guide for Patients and Carers*. London: Brain and Spine Foundation.

Brain and Spine Foundation (2005b) *Recovering from Sub-Arachnoid Haemorrhage: A Guide for Patients and Carers*. London: Brain and Spine Foundation.

Broks, P. (2003) *Into the Silent Land*. London: Atlantic Books.

Buchanan, K.M., Elias, L.J. and Goplen, G.B. (2000) 'Differing perspectives on outcome after subarachnoid haemorrhage: the patient, the relative and the neurosurgeon', *Neurosurgery*, 46(4): 831–40.

Butler, G. and Hope, T. (1995) *Manage your Mind: The Mental Fitness Guide*. Oxford: Oxford University Press.

Carver, C.S. (1997) 'You want to measure coping but your protocol's too long: consider the Brief COPE', *International Journal of Behavioral Medicine*, 9: 92–100.

Cedzich, C. and Roth, A. (2005) 'Neurological and psychosocial outcome after a subarachnoid haemorrhage and the Hunt and Hess scale as a predictor of clinical outcome', *Zentralblatt für Neurochirurgie*, 66(3): 112–18.

Collett, A., Kent, W. and Swain, S. (2006) 'The role of a telephone helpline in provision of patient information', *Nursing Standard*, 20(32): 41–4.

DiCiccio-Bloom, B. and Crabtree, B.F. (2006) 'The qualitative research interview', *Medical Education*, 40: 314–21.

Didion, J. (2006) *The Year of Magical Thinking*. London: Harper Perennial.

Different Strokes (2007) *Work After Stroke*. Milton Keynes: Different Strokes.

Down, K., Hughes, R., Sinha, A., Higginson, I. and Leigh, N. (2005) *Involving Users in Shaping Motor Neurone Disease Services*. York: Joseph Rowntree Foundation.

Ely, M., Vinz, R., Downing, M. and Anzul, M. (1997) *Writing Qualitative Research: Living by Words*. London: Falmer Press.

Enevoldson, T.P. (2004) 'Recreational drugs and their neurological consequences', *Neurology, Neurosurgery and Psychiatry*, 75: 9–15.

Etherington, K. (2002) 'Working together: editing a book as narrative research methodology', *Counselling and Psychotherapy Research*, 3(2): 167–76.

Eysenbach, G., Powell, J., Englesakis, M., Rizo, C. and Stern, A. (2004) 'Health-related virtual communities and electronic support groups: systematic review of the effects of online peer to peer interactions', *British Medical Journal*, 328: 1166.

Foulkes, L. (2004) *Subarachnoid Haemorrhage*. Southampton: Wessex Neurological Centre.

Frankl, V. (1959) *Man's Search for Meaning*. New York/London: Pocket Books.

Gilbert, P. and Irons, C. (2005) 'Focused therapies and compassionate mind training for shame and self-attacking', in P. Gilbert (ed.) *Compassion: Conceptualisations, Research and Use in Psychotherapy*. London: Routledge, pp. 263–325.

Gillen, G. (2005) 'Positive consequences of surviving a stroke', *American Journal of Occupational Therapy*, 59(3): 346.

Grant, J. (2006) 'Lost and found: a personal account of trauma and healing narratives'. Presentation, 'Health, Illness and Representation': Fourth Annual Meeting of the Association for Medical Humanities UK, 4–5 September, King's College, London.

Guardian (2007) 'A working life: the neurosurgeon'. *Work* supplement, p.3, 24 February.

Hackett, M.L. and Anderson, C.S. (2000) 'Health outcomes one year after subarachnoid haemorrhage: an international population-based study', *Neurology*, 55(5): 658–62.

Hager, K. and Ziegler, K. (1998) 'Stages in coping after stroke', *Zeitschrift für Gerontologie und Geriatrie*, 31(1): 9–15.

Hamedani, A.G., Wells, C.K., Brass, L.M., Kernan, W.N., Viscoli, C.M., Maraire, J.N., Aswad, I.A. and Horwitz, R.I. (2001) 'A quality of life instrument for young haemorrhagic stroke patients', *Stroke*, March: 687–96.

Hardey, M. (2002) '"The story of my illness": personal accounts of illness on the internet', *Health: An Interdisciplinary Journal for the Social Study of Health, Illness and Medicine*, 6(1): 31–46.

Herman, J.L. (1994) *Trauma and Recovery*. London: Pandora.

Hop, J.W., Rinkel, G.J.E., Algra, A. and van Gjin, J. (1998) 'Quality of life in patients and partners after aneurysmal subarachnoid haemorrhage', *Stroke*, 29: 798–804.

Hutchinson, G.F. and Baillie, M.B. (1932) 'A case of subarachnoid haemorrhage with recovery', *Canadian Medical Association Journal*, 27(5): 509–12.

Hütter, B.O., Gilsbach, J.M. and Kreitschmann, I. (1995) 'Quality of life and cognitive deficits after subarachnoid haemorrhage', *British Journal of Neurosurgery*, 9(4): 465–75.

Jarvis, A. (2002) 'Recovering from subarachnoid haemorrhage: patients' perspective', *British Journal of Nursing*, 11(22): 1430–37.

Jarvis, A. and Talbot, L. (2004) 'Multiprofessional follow-up of patients after subarachnoid haemorrhage', *British Journal of Nursing*, 13(21): 1262–7.

Kirkness, C.J., Thompson, J.M., Ricker, B.A., Newell, D.W., Dikmen, S. and Mitchell, P.H. (2002) 'The impact of aneurysmal subarachnoid haemorrhage on functional outcome', *Journal of Neuroscience Nursing*, 34(3): 134–41.

Kirwilliam, S. and Sheldrick, R. (2005) *Managing Fatigue Following Acquired Brain Injury*. Salford: Brain and Spine Injury Charity.

Lapotaire, J. (2003) *Time Out of Mind*. London: Virago.

Larner, S. (2005) 'Common psychological challenges for patients with newly acquired disability', *Nursing Standard*, 19(28): 33–9.

Leary, M.R., Tate, E.B., Adams, C.E., Allen, A.B. and Hancock, J. (2007) 'Self-compassion and reactions to unpleasant self-relevant events: the implications of treating oneself kindly', *Personality and Social Psychology*, 92(5): 887–904.

Lindsay, K.W. and Bone, I. (1997) *Neurology and Neurosurgery Illustrated. Section IV*. Edinburgh: Churchill Livingstone.

Linley, P.A. and Joseph, S. (2002) 'Posttraumatic growth', *Counselling and Psychotherapy*, February: 14–17.

McCrum, R. (1998) *My Year Off: Rediscovering Life After a Stroke.* London: Picador.

McKenna, P., Willison, J.R. and Neil-Dwyer, G. (1989) 'Recovery after subarachnoid haemorrhage', *British Medical Journal*, 299: 485–7.

Mayo Clinic (2005) 'Resilience: build skills to endure hardship'. MayoClinic.com. Accessed 10.11.2007.

Mezue, W., Mathew, B., Draper, P. and Watson, R. (2004) 'The impact of care on carers of patients treated for aneurysmal subarachnoid haemorrhage', *British Journal of Neurosurgery*, 18(2): 135–7.

Moore, A.D. and Stambrook, M. (1992) 'Coping strategies and locus of control following traumatic brain injury: relationship to long-term outcome', *Brain Injury*, 6(1): 89–94.

Morris, P.G. (2001) 'Long-term neuropsychological outcome following subarachnoid haemorrhage or traumatic brain injury'. PhD thesis, Stirling University.

Morris, P.G., Wilson, J.T. and Dunn, L.T. (2004) 'Anxiety and depression after spontaneous subarachnoid haemorrhage', *Neurosurgery*, 54(1): 47–54.

National Institute for Clinical Excellence (NICE, 2005) *Coil Embolisation of Ruptured Intracranial Aneurysms.* London: NICE.

Nochi, M. (1998) 'Loss of self: a narrative study on people with traumatic brain injuries', *Dissertation Abstracts International, Section B*, 58(12-B), June.

Nochi, M. (2000) 'Reconstructing self-narratives in coping with traumatic brain injury', *Social Science and Medicine*, 51: 1795–1804.

Nursing Times (2005) 'Subarachnoid haemorrhage', *Nursing Times*, 101(2): 30. No author cited.

Office of Communication (OFCOM, 2007) *Digital Progress Report.* London: OFCOM.

Ogden, J. (2000) *Health Psychology: A Textbook*, 2nd edn. Maidenhead: Open University Press.

Ogden, J.A., Utley, T. and Mee, E.W. (1997) 'Neurological and psychosocial outcome 4 to 7 years after subarachnoid hemorrhage [sic]', *Neurosurgery*, 41(1): 25–34.

Orbach, S. (1999) *Towards Emotional Literacy.* London: Virago.

Osborn, C. (1998) *Over my Head: A Doctor's Own Story of Head Injury from the Inside Looking Out.* Kansas City: Andrews McMeel.

Parkes, C.M (1998) *Bereavement: Studies of Grief in Adult Life*, 3rd edn. Harmondsworth: Penguin.

Pennebaker, J.W., Kiecolt-Glaser, J.K. and Glaser, J. (1988) 'Disclosure of traumas and immune function: health implications for psychotherapy', *Consulting and Clinical Psychology*, 56: 239–45.

Pobereskin, L.H. (2001) 'Incidence and outcome of subarachnoid haemorrhage: a retrospective population based study', *Neurology, Neurosurgery and Psychiatry*, 70: 340–43.

Powell, J., Kitchen, N., Heslin, J. and Greenwood, R. (2002) 'Psychosocial outcomes at three and nine months after good neurological recovery from aneurysmal subarachnoid haemorrhage: predictors and prognosis', *Neurology, Neurosurgery and Psychiatry*, 72: 722–81.

Powell, J., Kitchen, N., Heslin, J. and Greenwood, R. (2004) 'Psychosocial outcomes at 18 months after good neurological recovery from aneurysmal subarachnoid haemorrhage', *Neurology, Neurosurgery and Psychiatry*, 75: 1119–24.

Powell, T. (2004) *Head Injury: A Practical Guide*, 2nd edn. Bicester: Speechmark with Headway.

Pritchard, C., Foulkes, L., Lang, D.A. and Neil-Dwyer, G. (2001) 'Psychosocial outcomes for patients and carers after aneurysmal subarachnoid haemorrhage', *British Journal of Neurology*, 15(6): 456–63.

Pritchard, C., Foulkes, L., Lang, D. and Neil-Dwyer, N. (2004) 'Cost-benefit analysis of an integrated approach to reduce psychosocial trauma following neurosurgery compared with standard care: two-year prospective comparative study of enhanced specialist liaison nurses service for aneurysmal subarachnoid haemorrhage (ASAH) patients and carers', *Surgical Neurology*, 62: 17–27.

Raine, N.V. (2000) *After Silence: Rape & My Journey Back*. London: Virago.

Rimmon-Kenan, S. (2005) 'What can narrative therapy learn from illness narratives?' Literature and Medicine lecture series, King's College London, 28 May.

Sacks, O. (1986) *A Leg To Stand On*. London: Picador.

Scott, C.R. (2006) 'Coping skills after a subarachnoid haemorrhage: a quality of life study'. Unpublished dissertation, MSc Applied Psychology, Brunel University.

Sheldrick, R., Tarrier, N., Berry, E. and Kincey, J. (2006) 'Post-traumatic stress disorder and illness perceptions over time following myocardial infarction and subarachnoid haemorrhage', *British Journal of Health Psychology*, 11: 387–400.

Stone, S.D. (2007) *A Change of Plans: Women's Stories of Hemorrhagic Stroke*. Toronto: Sumach Press.

Taylor, S. (1998) *Coping Strategies*. John D. and Catherine T. MacArthur Research Network on Socioeconomic Status and Health. www.macses.ucsf.edu/Research/Psychosocial/notebook/coping.html. Accessed 21.02.07.

Tschudin, V. (1997) *Counselling for Loss and Bereavement*. London: Baillière Tindall.

US National Cancer Institute (2007) www.cancer.gov/cancertopics/pdq/supportivecare/spirituality/patient. Accessed 20.11.2007.

Van Gjin, J., Kerr, R.S. and Rinkel, G.J. (2007) 'Subarachnoid haemorrhage', *Lancet*, 306–18.

Vanistendael, S. (1996) *Growth in the Muddle of Life. Resilience: Building on People's Strengths*, 2nd edn. Geneva: International Catholic Child Bureau.

Vega, C., Kwoon, J.V. and Lavine, S.D. (2002) 'Intercranial aneurysms: current evidence and clinical practice', *American Family Physician*, 66(4): 601–8.

Wallcraft, J. (2002) 'Turning towards recovery: a study of personal narratives of mental health crisis and breakdown'. PhD dissertation, South Bank University, London.

Ward, M. (2001) 'Jigsaw', *The Friend*, 24 August: 12.

Wermer, M.J., Kool, H., Albrecht, K.W. and Rinkel, G.J. (2007) 'Subarachnoid haemorrhage treated with clipping: long-term effects on employment, relationships, personality and mood', *Neurosurgery*, 60(1): 91–7.

Wertheimer, A. (2001) *A Special Scar: The Experiences of People Bereaved by Suicide*, 2nd edn. London: Routledge.

Wessex Neurological Centre (2007) *Our Story: Patient Experiences of Subarachnoid Haemorrhage*. DVD, 33 mins. Southampton: Southampton General Hospital.

INDEX

acceptance 209–11
Adams, C.E. 212, 248
adjustment 209–11
advice 38, 83–6
ageing and recovery 54–5
Albrecht, K.W .182, 183, 192, 251
Algra, A. 42, 116, 159, 220, 226, 248
Allen, A.B. 212, 248
Al-Shahi, R. 35, 36, 92, 99, 246
Anderson, C.S. 182, 248
Andrew: on ageing 54; biographical
details 240; on children 161; on
cognitive difficulties 121; on
control 147; on counselling 101; on
early recovery 73, 75; on
employment 185, 187–8, 189–90,
191–2; on fatigue 110; on going out
174; on hidden difficulties 62; on
neurosurgery care 70; on peer
support 89; on post-haemorrhage
changes 220, 230, 224, 233, 234; on
reasons for interview 45; on sexual
activity 159; on strategies for
recovery 201, 207–8 218; on
subarachnoid haemorrhage 33, 34;
on support groups 93; on
swimming 178; on written account
49–50, 51
aneurysms 33, 35, 54, 244
anger 141–4
angiogram 244
Anthony, W.A. 52–3, 246
anxiety 38, 39, 74, 85, 130–5
Anzul, M. 45, 247
aphasia 244
arachnoid 244

arteriovenous malformation (AVM)
35, 42
artery 244
Aswad, I.A. 42, 248
attention 117, 122–4
Ausman, J.I. 37, 38, 135, 246

Baillie, M.B. 36, 248
BBC 27, 246
behindthegray.net 90
Beristain, X. 37, 38, 135, 246
berry aneurysms *see* aneurysms
Berry, E. 63, 85, 250
blame *see* self-blame
Blastland, M. 2, 246
BMJ (*British Medical Journal*) 92,
246
Bone, I. 33, 35, 248
Boss, P. 215, 246
Brain and Spine Foundation 6, 33,
35, 36, 40, 55, 58, 84, 90, 104, 108,
112, 114, 115, 116, 117, 120, 124,
125, 128, 148, 159, 170, 172, 176,
177, 178, 182, 183, 213, 214, 237,
241, 246
Brain and Spine Injury Charity
(BASIC) 241, 243
Brain Aneurysm Foundation 241
Brain Aneurysm Self-Help (BASH)
243
brain, meaning of: for survivors 25–6;
for neurosurgeons 26–7
Brass, L.M. 42, 248
Brian: biographical details 240; on
cognitive difficulties 119, 120; on
employment 185–6, 188; on

services 100; on early days of
recovery 72; on employment 196;
on financial effects 198; on friends
169; on GPs 97; on hidden
difficulties 60–1; on individual
recovery 53; on internet 91; on lack
of memory of hospital stay 80; on
onset of haemorrhage 64; on post-
haemorrhage changes 232–3; on
self-confidence 138–9; on sleep
disturbance 113; on socialising 173;
on spouses 158–9; on strategies for
recovery 215; on support groups
94; on timescales of recovery 56
self, changed view of 231–4
self-blame 148–50
self-compassion 211–12
self-confidence 39, 108, 137–40
self-esteem *see* self-confidence
self-image *see* self-confidence
sensory effects 103–16
sexual activity after haemorrhage
159–60
Sheldrick, R. 63, 85, 108, 112, 113,
125, 248, 250
Shirley: biographical details 240; on
cognitive functioning 117; on post-
haemorrhagic changes 238; on
spouses 155–6; on driving 177; on
written account 50
Short-term memory *see* memory
shunt 60, 245
Sinha, A. 90, 247
sleep disturbance 112–13
smell, sense of 115
socialising 170–4
specialist units *see* neurosurgery
units
specialist nurses 38, 94–6
speech *see* language difficulties
speech therapy 99, 100, 101, 245
spirituality and religion 219, 230–1
sports and exercise 177–9
spouses and partners 155–61
Stambrook, M. 202, 249
Stark, J.L. 37, 38, 135, 246
Stern, A. 90, 247
Stone, S.D. 28, 29, 250
stroke, haemorrhagic 26, 29, 42, 57,
59 87, 108, 174, 178, 187, 245

Stroke Association 90, 242
Subarachnoid Haemorrhage Support
Group (Newcastle) 243
Subarachnoid Haemorrhage Support
Group (Wessex) 243
subarachnoid haemorrhage:
definitions 33; descriptions 33–4;
causes 35; incidence 35; age 35, 54;
gender 35, 54; risk factors 35–6;
diagnosis 36; treatment 36; survival
rates 36; outcomes 37–9
support 38, 39, 63, 83, 85, 86, 88, 89,
90–1, 92; *see also* support groups
support groups 38, 88, 89–90, 92–4,
243
survivors: interviews 41–8; reasons
for interview 45–8; written
accounts: 48–51
Swain, S. 85, 86, 247

Talbot, L. 69, 83, 96, 99, 248
Tania: on anxiety 134; biographical
details 240; on cognitive difficulties
118, 119; on community services
10; on early recovery 74, 75, 78; on
employment 188, 190, 193; on
families 154–5; on fatigue 109–10,
111; on friends 167; on humour
77–8; on meeting new people 174;
on post-haemorrhage changes 226,
231, 234; on reaction to diagnosis
65, 77; on reasons for interview 48;
on self-blame 149–50; on self-
confidence 137–8; on socialising
172–3; on specialist nurses 95; on
strategies for recovery 214, 215,
217; on Terson's syndrome 107; on
timescales of recovery 55, 56
Tarrier, N. 63, 85, 250
taste, sense of 115
Tate, E.B. 212, 248
Taylor, S. 202, 250
telephone helplines 84
television, watching 180–1
Terson's syndrome 107
Thompson, J.M. 83, 248
tiredness *see* fatigue
trauma 63–6, 222–3; *see also* post-
traumatic stress disorder
Tschudin, V. 220, 250